Medical Emergencies
Diagnosis and Management

Medical Emergencies
Diagnosis and Management

FOURTH EDITION

RICHARD ROBINSON

F.R.C.P.
formerly registrar to the Renal Unit, Guy's Hospital

ROBIN STOTT

M.A., F.R.C.P.
Consultant Physician, Lewisham Hospital

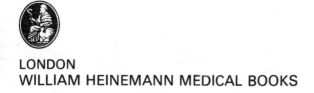

LONDON
WILLIAM HEINEMANN MEDICAL BOOKS

William Heinemann Medical Books,
22 Bedford Square, London WC1B 3HH

First published 1970
Second edition 1976
Reprinted with revisions 1977
Reprinted 1979
Third edition 1980
Reprinted 1981
Fourth edition 1983
Reprinted 1985, 1986, 1987

ISBN 0-433-28106-5

Typeset in VIP Times and Univers by
D. P. Media Limited, Hitchin, Hertfordshire
Printed in Great Britain by
Richard Clay Ltd, Bungay, Suffolk

Contents

Acknowledgements

Cardiovascular	— Graham Jackson & Paul Curry
Respiratory	— Tim Clark
G.I.	— Hermon Dowling
Renal	— Gwyn Williams
Endocrine	— Harry Keen
Neurology	— Richard Hughes
The Overdose	— Roy Goulding
General	— Gordon Jackson
Psychiatric and Social Problems	— Derry McDiarmid
Closed Head Injury	— Charles Polkey

Also the long suffering Mrs. Jean Smith and Mrs. Margaret Maw for their secretarial help.

Finally Alan Turner, whose criticism of the manuscript was invaluable.

Foreword

Every well-educated, newly appointed, Pre-Registration House Officer on the way to answer a call to deal with a medical emergency experiences the same anxieties about his ability to discharge his responsibilities when he gets there. One of my own strong memories is set in the Casualty Room at Johns Hopkins where I was acting as a Locum Intern: I recall a more senior colleague—long since an eminent Professor of Medicine—reaching up to take bottles of sterile glucose from the shelf as the comatose (hypoglycaemic) patient was wheeled in on the ambulance trolley. How could one, I wondered, ever match this speedy diagnostic acumen and authoritative management?

By experience, of course. But also through the knowledge accumulated by those who have faced the situation before and made important contributions by indicating the essential features to enquire about in the history, the signs to seek in the clinical examination, the laboratory measurements to order, and the first steps to take in management.

Emergencies are situations more than any others where one feels the drawbacks of our learning being divided into medical and surgical subjects, and further subdivided now into the organ specialities. House Officers have to assemble in a trice knowledge from many sources. In a way, this is the strength of the young Pre-Registration or Post-Registration House Officer: in this era of fast expanding knowledge he or she is, across the board, most up-to-date. But it demands a superb memory and a flexibility of thought given to very few of us.

Richard Robinson realised the need for a pocket manual about the essentials of the current diagnostic, therapeutic and management principles, to deal properly with medical emergencies. So he has written this book, to bring together information widely scattered in textbooks on many subjects. He has set things down on the assumption, correct I believe, that the users will be the graduates of the present era, *au fait* with current hospital facilities and modern drugs. He has aimed to help them by concise writing. Here and there, his approach may be regarded as didactic, but that hardly matters in the emergency situation. I therefore commend this book to all those young people into whose hands our most seriously ill emergencies first come, with my best wishes to them, for quick and accurate diagnosis, and to their patients, for speedy recovery!

W. J. H. Butterfield, OBE, DM, FRCP
Professor of Medicine, Guy's Hospital, London SE1

viii

Introduction to the previous editions

The aim of this book is still to supply a framework of knowledge into which the House Physician can fit his experience. Some of the facilities mentioned are not available in many hospitals. If by creating awareness of deficiencies patient care is improved, this book will be justified.

Since this book was first written we have become acutely aware of another dimension of its subject. The sobering fact is that the bulk of medical emergencies, which attract so much glamour and therefore money, talent and facilities, are preventable. This applies to each of the big four—coronary artery disease, cerebrovascular accidents, acute respiratory failure and overdoses. A moment's thought will show that the causes of each of these lie in the way we respond to our social and economic situation. The increasingly complex technology of medicine has been associated with the increasing isolation of its practitioners. This has led to a pre-empting by doctors of major areas of the patient's involvement with his disease. It is all too easy to treat patients in a life-threatening situation as a physiological preparation, and to overlook the fact that the patient and his family have lived with the roots of his disease, will probably continue to do so, and will have to live with its results.

Effective prevention of these conditions will probably only begin when the responsibility for health care is taken where it belongs—in the community. The effect of this aspect of treatment—which we have almost wholly ignored—will be far greater than the results obtained by the successful management of acute emergencies.

Introduction to the fourth edition

Despite our increasing years, and in one case baldness, we have maintained an active interest in and close exposure to emergency medicine. It is interesting to compare the material in the original edition of this book, published in 1970, with the present text. Some chapters such as a number in the endocrinological section have changed very little. Rapid changes in renal medicine had occurred just prior to 1970 but little in this field has since made an impact in the acute situation. The more mechanistic emergencies such as distressing pleural and pericardial effusions, pneumothorax, laryngeal obstruction and acute gastric dilatation still yield to the same relatively straightforward manoeuvres. Other chapters have changed beyond recognition. Our improved understanding of the pathophysiology of many varieties of shock have altered our therapeutic approach, the increasing complexity of cardiac arrhythmias has not faltered, and of course the advance of non-invasive imaging has made a major impact in the management of acute neurology. For this edition a new topic, that of closed head injury, has been introduced.

We must re-iterate the caveat that the immediacy of acute medicine should not blind any of us to the importance of prevention. Most of the emergencies detailed in this book would not have occurred if appropriate action had been taken to forestall the pathological processes which underlie much illness in the developed world today.

The increase in technology has done nothing to diminish the importance of our fallible clinical skills upon which we continue to rely not only in the diagnostic exercise but also in deciding when and how much to intervene. This decision may need to be taken relatively early in the course of events. It has become inevitable that the relative clinical independence enjoyed by many recently qualified doctors fifteen years ago is no longer in the best interests of his patient. Although more closely supervised now we hope that he will continue to find this book informative and reassuring.

CARDIOVASCULAR

Cardiac arrest

Before you ever have to deal with a cardiac arrest be prepared by:

(1) Knowing how to use the defibrillator.
(2) Knowing how to inflate the patient with 100% oxygen.

DIAGNOSIS

Cardiac arrest can be considered to have occurred if the carotid or femoral pulses are absent. Do not waste time trying to hear the heart.

MANAGEMENT

(1) Check the time.
(2) Put the patient on the floor—if not already on fracture boards—and start cardiac massage at about 60 compressions per minute. Effective cardiac massage produces a femoral pulse.
(3) Get someone to give mouth-to-mouth respiration (the aesthetics of this can be improved by laying a handkerchief over the face of the patient). Give 3–5 compressions to one inflation. It's neither necessary nor desirable to stop compressing the heart whilst your assistant inflates the chest.[5]
(4) Check that the anaesthetist and emergency trolley, ECG, or oscilloscope, and defibrillator have all been sent for.
(5) Get the bed out of the way—you will need space.
(6) Get a sucker. The patient will soon vomit if he has not already done so.
(7) Get a drip up. Use the needle you are most familiar with. A number 1 needle taped to the skin will do. Try the antecubital fossae first. Failing this, subclavian or, internal jugular puncture give rapid reliable access to the circulation. If you are not familiar with these techniques, expose the long saphenous vein at the ankle, and under direct vision insert the needle. Do not waste time doing a formal cut down however.
(8) Get a drip stand—or hang the bottle from the hooks in the curtain rail.

(9) Attach a giving set to a bottle of 8·4% bicarbonate. A nurse should do (6), (8) and (9) whilst you are doing (7).

(10) Run in 100 ml of 8·4% bicarbonate (i.e. 100 mmol of bicarbonate). Thereafter run in 60 ml every 15 minutes. Be careful; there is a tendency to give too much bicarbonate during an arrest.

(11) If the anaesthetist is not forthcoming insert the cuffed endotracheal tube yourself—size 9 or 10 for an average-sized adult. Re-aquaint yourself with this technique by practising after each unsuccessful cardiac arrest. The patient must not become hypoxic. If you have difficulty at first, stop every 15 seconds and re-inflate as in (3).

(12) Check that the tube is in the trachea by pressing the chest (and getting a puff back up the tube) or by blowing down the tube (and listening to the chest). Anchor it to the face by taping or strapping.

(13) Attach the patient to your source of oxygen supply and inflate once every five seconds—between every third or fourth chest compression.

(14) Deliver a 400 joule shock with the defibrillator as soon as it arrives. If the cardiac activity is ventricular fibrillation (VF) this may be life-saving. Delay—in order to establish the nature of the cardiac arrhythmia—lessens the chances of successfully provoking a return to sinus rhythm. Delivering a shock will do the patient no harm if the heart is in asystole.

Points to remember are:

(i) Straddle the electrodes across the heart—preferably one on the anterior chest wall and one on the posterior.

(ii) Do not get electrode jelly smeared across the skin between the electrodes—it will conduct current (Caution—KY jelly does not contain electrolytes and is less efficient).

(iii) Do not stand in puddles of blood or saline.

(iv) Ensure that the electrodes are smeared with fresh jelly at each attempt.

(v) Ensure that no one else is touching the patient or the bed.

(15) Attach the patient to an ECG or an oscilloscope as soon as possible. Machines in which the defibrillator paddles also act as ECG electrodes are now available.

(16) If ventricular fibrillation persists after three or four attempts at DC conversion.

    (i)   Give one or more of the following drugs intravenously:

        (a) Lignocaine 50 mg if VF is coarse or paroxysmal. Lignocaine should not be used if VF is of low amplitude.

        (b) Disopyramide 100 mg i.v.

    (ii) Now try and defibrillate again.

    (iii) If, after several attempts you are still unsuccessful, one or more of the following drugs are worth trying intravenously:

        (a) Phenytoin sodium 100 mg.

        (b) Magnesium sulphate 5–10 mmol of a 20% solution (6–12 ml).

        (c) Bretylium tosylate 5 mg/kg i.v. (followed by 100 mg i.m. hourly to a maximum of 2·0 g).

Should you successfully control VF, maintain a lignocaine infusion 2–4 mg/min for 24 hours.

Bad prognostic signs are:

    (i)   Steadily decreasing amplitude of fibrillation. The amplitude may be increased by giving calcium and adrenaline.[21,22]

    (ii) A tendency for DC shock to cause asystole.

(17) If the heart is in asystole try to restart a normal rhythm or at least VF.

    (i)   Give:

        (a) 10 ml of 1:10 000 adrenaline (or 1 ml of 1:1000 adrenaline).

        (b) 10 ml of 10% calcium gluconate—both intravenously.

    (ii) Wait for the heart to fibrillate and then defibrillate.

    (iii) If fibrillation does not occur within five minutes repeat the dose of adrenaline.

    (iv) If this is not successful give an intracardiac injection of 5 ml of 1:10 000 adrenaline together with 5 ml of 10%

calcium gluconate. Put a chest aspiration needle on your syringe and insert this in the 4th intercostal space, to the left of the midline. Push the needle in on suction until you withdraw blood. This should be from the heart and you can then inject the adrenaline directly into the chamber.

(v) Continue cardiac massage to pump the injection into the coronary arteries.

(18) If the heart is an atrial asystole with widely spread ineffectual ventricular beats, provoke ventricular fibrillation and defibrillate as above.

(19) Whilst (13) to (17) are going on, 10 to 15 minutes will have elapsed. By this time the patient should be reasonably pink. If he is not, consider the following:

(i) Efforts at ventilation are insufficient. The usual tendency is to underestimate the rate and depth of ventilation needed and it is sometimes salutory to measure the blood gases during a cardiac arrest.

(ii) The patient has inhaled masses of vomit. Suck this out through the endotracheal tube. If your resuscitation is subsequently successful remember to give high doses of corticosteroids as a prophylaxis to vomit induced 'shock lung' (see p. 83).

(iii) The endotracheal tube is past the carina and is in one main bronchus. Withdraw the tube slightly. Both (iii) and (vi) will give poor breath sounds with diminished movement on one side. If in doubt try (iii) first.

(iv) The patient has had a massive pulmonary embolus. The lungs will resist inflation.

(v) The oxygen supply has run out. You don't know when this occurred so carry on.

(vi) The patient has a pneumothorax (see p. 73).

(20) Other points to bear in mind are:

(i) The cause of the arrest: acute hypoxia, fits, upper airways obstruction, electrolyte disturbances such as hypo or hyperkalaemia, and digoxin poisoning, are potentially reversible. Severe brain injury, massive pulmonary emboli and ruptured aortic aneurysms are not.

(ii) Full recovery has been recorded after the pupils have

been fully dilated. This sign is not in itself a sufficient reason for stopping.

(iii) Do not forget cardiac tamponade (*see* p. 51). If due to a tense effusion it may be necessary to aspirate the pericardial space or if due to blood clot an emergency thoracotomy (at the bedside) is indicated. The heart may then be difibrillated directly using internal paddles. A thoracotomy may also have to be performed if you are not obtaining an adequate circulation for some other reason, e.g. regurgitant heart valves.

(iv) Finally— and more rapidly acquired with experience than you might think—try and keep a detached attitude. When the situation is under control—i.e. the drip is up, the patient is being inflated and the ECG or oscilloscope is running—get someone else to do the cardiac massage, step back and decide what you are going to do next and for how long you are going to continue.

Myocardial infarction[6,8,14,18]

DIAGNOSIS

(1) Myocardial infarction usually presents with a history of severe crushing retrosternal chest pain, often radiating to the neck and arms.

(2) However, it may present in a number of indirect ways, particularly in the elderly, for example:

    (i) Fainting, giddy turns, palpitations or 'collapse'.
    (ii) Acute left ventricular failure.
    (iii) Unexplained hypotension (commonly post-operative).
    (iv) A peripheral embolus.
    (v) A stroke (either due to (iii) or (iv)).
    (vi) Diabetic keto-acidosis.

(3) It is sometimes difficult to be sure that a myocardial infarction has not occurred. In such cases, the patient must be admitted for observation, and serial ECGs and cardiac enzymes done. The creatine phosphokinase (CPK) is particularly useful, as it invariably rises within the 12 hours after infarction. A rise in CPK due to other causes, e.g. intra-muscular injections, may be distinguished by assaying the MB CPK iso-enzyme, which is more prevalent in cardiac muscle. A normal ECG does not exclude the diagnosis of myocardial infarction. A proportion of these patients may have the pre-infarction syndrome (see p. 16).

MANAGEMENT

All patients must have either a drip or a heparinised canula (Venflon) inserted. Drugs must be given i.v. both for speed and because absorption by other routes is uncertain when perfusion is diminished. Then three things need urgent attention. In order of priority they are:

(1) **Pain Control**
Heroin 5 mg i.v. or morphine 10–15 mg i.v. (each with 50 mg cyclizine or 12·5 mg prochlorperazine one minute beforehand to

forestall vomiting) are still the drugs of choice. The new synthetic narcotic agents have no advantage over these two drugs. Pentazocine (Fortral) may cause a rise in pulmonary artery pressure and should not be used.

Under no circumstances withold these drugs from patients suffering from myocardial pain. If you are worried about the possibility of respiratory depression, monitor the blood gases and treat appropriately (q.v.). However, if necessary respiratory and circulatory depression due to narcotics can be counteracted by:

(i)   Naloxone $0\cdot4$–$1\cdot2$ mg i.v. in divided doses over 3 minutes.
(ii) Nalorphine 5–10 mg repeated to a dose of 40 mg, if you don't have naloxone.
(iii) Doxapram, by continuous infusion $1\cdot5$ mg/min to a maximum of $2\cdot5$ mg/min.

(2) **Arrythmias** must be treated (*see* p. 17). Bradycardia in the acute stage should be treated with atropine $0\cdot6$–$1\cdot2$ mg i.v.
(3) **Heart Failure**

(i)   This may be due to (1) or (2) above and should be treated appropriately. Otherwise impaired ventricular function results either from loss of functioning muscle, or mechanical disruption of the ventricular wall (VSD or rupture of the wall with tamponade) or valves (acute mitral regurgitation). Mechanical disruption usually occurs later in the course of the disease (2–10 days).
(ii) Invasive haemodynamic studies in normal subjects show that cardiac output is between $2\cdot2$–$4\cdot3$ litres/sq metre/min. If measured cardiac output falls below $2\cdot2$ litres/sq metre/min, clinical symptoms of poor perfusion (cool peripheries, hypotension, oliguria and a tendency toward mental confusion) are present. This is called pump failure. Similarly, normal pulmonary capillary wedge pressure (PCWP—an indirect measure of left atrial pressure) is below 18 mmHg. If the PCWP exceeds 25 mmHg the signs of pulmonary oedema develop (*see* p. 32); these are dyspnoea, added heart sounds, later inspiratory crackles on auscultation, and enlargement of the pulmonary veins, particularly to the upper lobe, on the chest x-ray, all this with or without radiological oedema. Heart failure and left

ventricular failure are therefore unhelpful terms since they may refer either to pulmonary oedema, or to the consequences of low cardiac output (pump failure), or both.

(iii) Haemodynamics studies in patients with myocardial infarction measuring cardiac output and pulmonary wedge pressure have shown that there are four groups of patients.[10]

Since the clinical picture correlates well with the haemodynamic findings (*see* (ii) above) we use the following clinical classification on which to build a rational approach to therapy.

Group	Clinical features	Haemodynamic characteristics	Average mortality
a	No pulmonary oedema	Normal PCWP (<18 mmHg)	1%
	Good perfusion	Normal cardiac output (>2·2 1/min)	
b	Pulmonary oedema	Raised PCWP (>25 mmHg)	10%
	Good perfusion	Normal cardiac output	
c	No pulmonary oedema Poor perfusion—pump failure	Normal PCWP Low cardiac output (<2·2 1/min)	20%
d	Pulmonary oedema Poor perfusion—pump failure	Raised PCWP Low cardiac output	60%

TREATMENT

Group a

(i) No specific therapy is required.

(ii) But therapy directed at reducing infarct size is being investigated.[7, 15]

The following are being used

(a) β-Blockers such as propranolol (as for pre-infarction syndrome) (*see* p. 16).

(b) Vasodilators, such as Na nitroprusside (*see* p. 38) or Trinitrin 1 mg orally two-hourly.[10, 14]

(c) Streptokinase, whose role in recanalisation of acutely blocked coronary arteries is under evaluation.[11]

Since group **a** have a good prognosis, the general acceptance of these approaches must await a clear demonstration of their value.

Group b

(i) A diuretic such as frusemide 40 mg i.v. is the best way of reducing pulmonary wedge pressure and relieving pulmonary congestion.

(ii) You should monitor the dose in accordance with your patient's response. Clinical improvement often precedes both radiological improvement and the disappearance of physical signs. An excessive diuresis can cause hypovolaemia, so bear this lag phenomenon in mind when adjusting diuretic doses. Conversely tachypnoea, as a result of decreased lung compliance, will precede the development of frank pulmonary oedema.

(iii) Digoxin. Do not use this routinely. In a situation of deteriorating failure, the therapy outlined under group **d** should be used.

Groups c and d

These two constitute the entity previously called 'cardiogenic shock'. Before embarking on therapy it is invaluable to have a Swan-Ganz catheter in place to measure pulmonary capillary wedge pressure; ideally cardiac output should also be measured. Central venous pressure should also be measured, but it is only an indirect, and hence frequently misleading, indication of left ventricular function. However, changes in CVP taken in conjunction with clinical observations can provide a basis on which to act (*see* p. 276).

Group c

It is mandatory to exclude hypovolaemia in this group. Hypovolaemia after infarction is more common than generally appreciated and may be explained in some—though not all—patients by the prolonged periods of anorexia, vomiting or sweating that accompany infarction. Therefore:

(i) Give i.v. dextran 70 made in 5% dextrose, or plasma, or albumin, until the PCWP approaches 18 mmHg or until the CVP approaches the upper normal range without the development of tachypnoea.

(ii) If hypovolaemia has been treated or excluded, pump failure may be a consequence of an inadequate heart rate in the presence of a low fixed stroke volume. Treat sinus bradycardia with atropine and heart block or slow atrial fibrillation with a pacemaker set at 90–100 beats per minute. Remember that atrial transport may contribute up to 30% of cardiac output so that pacing of a refractory sinus bradycardia may achieve little improvement in output. It is better to use isoprenaline or dopamine (*see* below).

(iii) For persistent pump failure with an adequate rate and volume, proceed as for group **d**.

Group d

Many of these patients will die, but treatment may occasionally be gratifyingly successful. Rational treatment is based on the idea that the ischaemic myocardium will improve in function if oxygen delivery is increased or oxygen consumption reduced. Increasing delivery is achieved by increasing coronary artery flow. Reducing consumption is achieved primarily by reducing left ventricular afterload (in effect reducing the peripheral resistance). Reducing left ventricular pre-load (in effect normalising the pulmonary capillary wedge pressure) whilst not directly reducing consumption, will relieve the heart of an additional burden, and is a desirable objective.

If a useful reduction in consumption is to be achieved, reduction in the pre-load and after load has to be effected without increasing the heart rate much above 100 beats/minute, the rate above which the law of diminishing returns sets in. Vasodilators which act on both veins and arteries, but which do not have a chronotropic effect, are the agents best suited to achieve this desired reduction in oxygen consumption. Although vasodilation may marginally improve oxygen delivery, only intra-aortic balloon pumping (*see* (vi) below) has a favourable effect on supply and consumption. Inotropic agents increase demand more than supply, and we therefore regard vasodilators as the first line in treatment. Therefore, use:

(i) NaNitroprusside 0·5—10 μg/kg/min. Nitroprusside has a half-life of 2–5 minutes. It may cause profound hypotension[14] (though, paradoxically this is less likely to happen with iller patients). Careful titration of the dose using intra-arterial monitoring is therefore mandatory. We use a short cannula—usually an 18 G Venflon in the radial artery. Electronic monitoring is ideal, but an anaeroid (Tychos) gauge or even direct manometry using a manometer line strung up on a tall drip stand may be satisfactory. If you cannot use nitroprusside for lack of intra-arterial monitoring use:

(ii) Salbutamol, 3–20 μg/min. This acts primarily as a vasodilator and may be managed using routine reading of CVP and BP.

(iii) If poor perfusion persists (hourly urine output and toe temperature are the best clinical guides to this) then add (or change to)

    (a) Dopamine 2–10 μg/kg/min. In this dose range dopamine has little overall effect on systemic resistance; however, the preferential increase in renal flow makes it the catecholamine of choice.[16]

    (b) Isoprenaline 0·5–10 μg/min.

    (c) Dobutamine 2·5–10·0 μg/kg/min.

(iv) Digitalisation is a form of inotropic support which seems to have little theoretical advantage over the catecholamines. However, some clinicians feel unhappy if their patients are not digitalised in these circumstances, in which case a quick acting compound with a short half-life seems preferable. We use oubaine, which acts within 5–10 minutes, has its peak effect within 0·5–2 hours, and which has a half-life of 21 hours (digoxin's half-life is 36 hours). The starting dose of oubaine is 500 μg i.v., repeated at four-hourly intervals as necessary, to a maximum of 2·0 mg in 24 hours.

(v) Infuse 500 ml of 20% glucose, containing 39 mmol KCl and 20 units of soluble insulin (GIK) over 6 hours. This is said to improve myocardial contractility, but its use is controversial. This same regime may also be helpful in the 'sick cell syndrome'. Here, the sodium pump, which is responsible for the extrusion of sodium from cells, falters. The intracellular sodium rises as the extracellular sodium falls, and the altered ionic milieu causes widespread, and often disastrous, metabolic consequences. The sick cell syndrome often occurs as a terminal event in many serious illnesses, and so the above regime is only occasionally helpful.

(vi) Balloon pumping is theoretically the most potent intervention in these circumstances. If balloon pumping is available it must be used early; it is unlikely to be of any value in patients who have had the signs of pump failure for longer than 4 hours. It is of particular value when combined with surgery in the management of mechanical disruption of the ventricle.

Having put in a venous line and treated pain, arrhythmias and failure, bear in mind the following important factors in all patients.

(1) Anxiety. Many patients are already aware of their diagnosis and it provides for them a most potent intimation of mortality. Reassurance is of paramount importance, if necessary supported by diazepam 5–10 mg i.v. or 2–5 mg t.d.s. orally. Lorazepam 1–4 mg i.v. or 1–2 mg t.d.s. orally is a possibly better alternative sedative.

Give oxygen (40%) via an MC mask as even patients with minor infarcts may have a low Pao_2.

(2) Consider anticoagulants.[9, 21, 57] 5000 units heparin s.c. eight-hourly started within 8 hours of the infarction, prevents thrombo-embolism as effectively as conventional full anticoagulation. In addition, hypertension and peptic ulceration are not contra-indications to this regime. Full anticoagulation with i.v. heparin may be given either intermittently 10 000 units six-hourly, or, preferably by continuous infusion using a suitable pump. In this case start with 10 000 units six-hourly, but monitor the dose to keep the partial thromboplastin time (PTT) between 2–4 times normal.[52] With either of the above regimes, we suggest continuing heparin for 5 days. In the evening of the last 3 days give warfarin 9 mg orally. On the sixth day, switch to warfarin exclusively, with the dosage monitored by the prothrombin time. Remember that heparin is inactivated by dextrose, only infuse it in normal saline.

(3) Streptokinase[19] (230 000 i.u. initially and then 100 000 i.u. hourly for 24 hours) has been tried but generally without obvious benefit.

(4) Check the blood sugar—many patients with an infarct get

stress-induced hyperglycaemia, and raised sugar may predispose towards arrhythmias. Persistent hyperglycaemia should be treated either with oral hypoglycaemic agents, or more satisfactorily in the acute situation, with an i.v. insulin infusion (*see* p. 134) commencing at a dose of 2 units/hour. There is some evidence that careful control of the blood sugar after infarction improves the prognosis.

(5) Routine lignocaine prophylaxis[36, 38]—some people advocate routine lignocaine prophylaxis, using an initial dose of 100 mg i.v. then using 1, 2 or 3 mg/min for 48 hours following the infarction. The benefits of this are still controversial so we do not routinely use prophylactic lignocaine.

Pre-infarction syndrome

DIAGNOSIS

The pre-infarction syndrome consists of:

    (i)   Recurrent angina at rest.
    (ii)   Increasing angina not relieved by trinitrin.
    (iii) Variable and transient ECG changes.
    (iv) Normal enzyme levels.

About one in seven of these patients will progress to myocardial infarction in the short term if left untreated.

MANAGEMENT

(1) Anxiety and pain should be managed as for myocardial infarction.
(2) Give nitrites (GTN by bedside) and isorbide dinitrite 5–10 mg six-hourly.[24]
(3) Give propranolol[26] in a dose sufficient either to stop pain or to reduce the pulse rate below 50 beats/min. Start at 20 mg four-hourly (orally) and increase as necessary.
(4) Give nifedipine 10–20 mg three times a day in addition for persisting unstable angina.
(5) Anticoagulants may not prevent the development of infarction but are indicated on the same basis as in myocardial infarction.
(6) Patients whose symptoms persist despite the above and in whom there is no evidence of infarction should be considered for coronary arteriogram with a view to coronary artery surgery. Intra-aortic balloon pump assist before surgery should be considered.[25] Streptokinase[11] in this situation is also being evaluated.

Cardiac arrhythmias

This may be supraventricular arising from the atria (atrial) or from around the A-V node (junctional) or ventricular (arising below the A-V node). They cause too rapid a heart action (tachycardia), occasional irregularities in rhythm (ectopics) or too slow a heart action (bradycardia). Also included in this section are arrhythmias where there is an abnormal relationship between atrial and ventricular contraction.

Arrhythmias are encountered most commonly after myocardial infarction. They may occur terminally after a period of hypotension and congestive cardiac failure in which case they are usually resistant to treatment (so-called secondary arrhythmias). However, they may also occur as a temporary disturbance in a heart capable of maintaining an adequate circulation. It is in this group, the primary arrhythmias, that treatment may be life-saving.

Arrhythmias may be potentiated or even caused by the following:

(1) Pain and anxiety—always ask your patient specifically about the presence of pain, he may be stoical.
(2) Hypoxia (which is often impossible to detect clinically).
(3) Acidosis.
(4) Hypo or hyperkalaemia.
(5) Hypo or hypercalcaemia.
(6) Sick cell syndrome (the escape of Na^+ into the K^+ out of cells is potentially reversible with glucose, K^+ and insulin (*see* p. 13).

Correction of these abnormalities may stop the arrhythmia and will certainly make it more amenable to treatment.

Supraventricular arrhythmias

Atrial Ectopics (Fig. 1)

These may be caused by digoxin and catecholamines. They may occur in otherwise normal hearts, especially during pregnancy. They may occur after myocardial infarction when they are usually benign, but may occasionally herald atrial tachycardia or fibrillation. In this situation, as at other times, they are not treated, other than by reassurance and, if necessary, mild sedation.

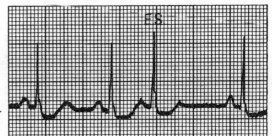

Fig. 1.
Supraventricular extrasystole. The small pointed P wave can be seen deforming the preceding T wave.

E.S. = extrasystole.

Supraventricular tachycardia

(1) Sinus tachycardia comes on gradually, its rate is affected by posture, exercise, atropine, and is usually below 150 beats/min. There is always an underlying cause such as LVF, anxiety, fever or hypoxia, which should be looked for and treated as necessary. It needs to be differentiated from:

(2) Paroxysmal tachycardia (Fig. 2) which comes on abruptly. Its rate (usually >150 beats/min) is unaffected by any of the above but may be terminated by carotid sinus massage. This may be caused by digoxin, a factor which profoundly influences its treatment.

    If the patient is not on digoxin, you can:

    (i)   Do nothing, if there is no evidence of failure, and the patient tells you that his attacks are shortlived.

    (ii)   Intense vagal stimulation may control this arrhythmia. Traditionally, carotid massage is used to evoke this

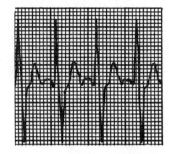

Fig. 2. *Supraventricular tachycardia*. The P wave can be clearly seen preceding each QRS complex.

response. The carotid sinus is level with the upper border of the thyroid cartilage. Press it firmly against the vertebral transverse process with a thumb and rub slowly half-an-inch up and down the artery. Only massage one side at a time. A newer approach is to make use of the 'diving response', which can be induced clinically by placing an ice bag on your patients face.[28]

(iii) The treatment of choice which is nearly always successful is *synchronised* DC reversion. This is carried out with an anaesthetist who gives a short acting anaesthetic (thiopentone 100–500 mg i.v. or ketamine—a bolus of 2 mg/kg given i.v. over 60 seconds gives 15 min anaesthesia). Ventilatory equipment should be available in case a temporary period of apnoea occurs. Give the shock observing the usual precautions (*see* p. 4) starting at 100 joules and increasing the stimulus by 50 joules until 400 joules are reached. If this is ineffective, try placing one 'paddle' on the patient's back behind the heart and one in front.

(iv) If DC reversion is either not available or not considered desirable, the following drugs may be useful:

(a) Verapamil 10 mg i.v.[29] This should not be used if any other anti-arrhythmic drug has been given before it, or if the patient is in shock, as it may cause irreversible asystole. It is emerging as the drug of choice in S.V.T.s however.

(b) Assuming your patient is not already on digoxin, a cardiac glycoside, such as oubaine, may be used (*see* p. 13).

(c) Try carotid sinus massage or a facial cold shock again after (a) and (b).

(d) Amiodarone 5 mg/kg infused over 10 minutes through a long intracatheter may be tried. If this is successful it may be continued as a continuous infusion; 600–1200 mg over 24 hours.

(e) All the drugs in (a), (b) and (d) above should be given slowly to minimise any adverse circulatory effects.

Atrial flutter (Fig. 3)

This may occur after myocardial infarction and with cardiomyopathies, ASD and systemic infections. It is not, unlike atrial fibrillation, associated with mitral stenosis or thyrotoxicosis. The atrium 'flutters' at an average rate of 300 beats/min. As the ventricles cannot respond at this rate there is always some degree of 'block' which may vary (Fig. 3).

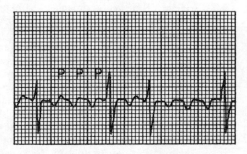

Fig. 3. *Atrial flutter.* The first three flutter waves are marked 'P'. The ventricles respond at a varying 1:2–1:3 ratio.

(1) Treatment of choice is DC reversion.
(2) Failing this, digitalise the patient. This may cause a reversion to sinus rhythm, or progression to atrial fibrillation.
(3) Verapamil, disopyramide or practolol may be given as for atrial tachycardia.

Atrial fibrillation and flutter fibrillation (Figs. 4 & 5)

(1) Are for practical purposes the same thing.
(2) The most common cause is ischaemic heart disease, but it also occurs after myocardial infarction, and in association with mitral valve disease, thyrotoxicosis, sub-acute bacterial endocarditis, atrial septal defect, constrictive pericarditis and after thoracotomy.

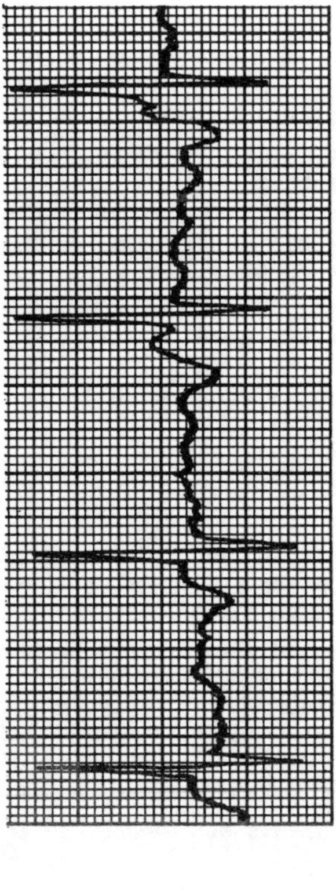

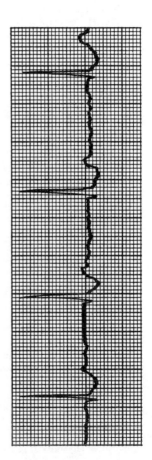

Fig. 4. *Atrial flutter fibrillation.* Coarse atrial activity is seen linking each QRS complex.

Fig. 5. *Atrial fibrillation.* Small amplitude atrial activity links each QRS complex.

(3) If the ventricular rate is sufficiently fast to cause cardiac failure the treatment of choice is digitalisation—combined if necessary with diuretics and oxygen (see pp. 11 and 14 respectively). Continue that dose of digoxin which maintains the ventricular rate between 70 and 80 beats/min.

(4) If the patient is severely distressed verapamil i.v. may be used whilst awaiting the effect of digoxin. Give 10 mg initially. If after 5 minutes there has been a response, but an incomplete one, a further 10 mg i.v. may be given once.

(5) DC reversion is unlikely to succeed if longstanding coronary artery disease is present, but should be considered electively after treatment of, for example, mitral stenosis or thyrotoxicosis (see p. 155).

Sinus bradycardia

Sinus bradycardia may occur with vasovagal attacks, intracranial hypertension, myxoedema (see p. 153) and in athletes in training. It is occasionally caused by β-adrenergic blocking agents, ganglion blocking hypotensive agents (e.g. guanethidine—especially when combined with digoxin) and by digoxin itself.

Bradycardia may also cause all the signs of severe cardiovascular collapse when it occurs after inferior myocardial infarction.[22] In this situation give atropine 0·6 mg i.v. Repeat this dose if there is no effect within five minutes. Response is usually prompt and gratifying. Atropine may cause ventricular fibrillation, urinary retention and glaucoma, and it is unwise to give more than 2·4 mg. Isoprenaline (see p. 245) may be used if atropine fails and treatment is deemed necessary.

Sinus arrest (Fig. 6)

May be caused by many of the anti-arrhythmic drugs, hyperkalaemia, excessive vagal tone, and myocardial infarction. Short periods of sinus inactivity may progress to permanent sinus arrest and if they occur a transvenous intracardiac pacemaker should be passed urgently.[37] Prior to this sinus rhythm may be restored by a sharp precordial blow or by atropine 0·6 mg i.v.

Junctional

Junctional rhythms represent the action of a built in pacemaker

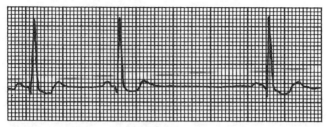

Fig. 6. *Sinus arrest*. After the second beat there is a temporary delay in sinus activity before the third beat is initiated.

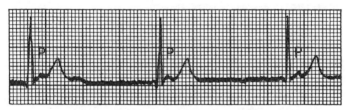

Fig. 7. *Junctional rhythm*. The P wave of each beat is clearly seen deforming the ST segment.

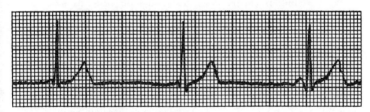

Fig. 8. *Junctional rhythm*. The P wave is seen immediately preceding each QRS complex.

which takes over as a result of sinus node dysfunction—the commonest causes of which are digoxin toxicity, myocardial infarction and myocarditis (Figs. 7 and 8). If the rate is sufficiently slow to cause cardiac failure, atropine 0·6 mg i.v. may provoke the sinus node to return at the normal rate. Failing this isoprenaline (*see* p. 245) may encourage acceleration of the junctional rhythms. Junctional tachycardias are treated as for their atrial counterparts (Fig. 9).

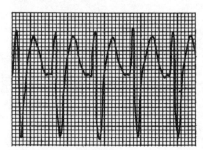

Fig. 9. *Junctional tachycardia*. A small P wave is seen immediately preceding each wide QRS complex.

VENTRICULAR ARRHYTHMIAS

Ventricular ectopics (Fig. 10)

Occur in myocardial infarction and in cardiomyopathies or as a result of digoxin toxicity.

(1) They may herald ventricular tachycardia or fibrillation (death, although sudden, is not always unannounced) if:

    (i)   They interrupt the T wave or ST segment of the preceding complex (in technical terms, if their coupling interval is short).

    (ii)   They are of multifocal origin.

    (iii) They are frequent (more than 10/min).

    (iv) More than two occur in succession.

They may be provoked by pain, hypoxia or hypocalcaemia. If treatment of these circumstances does not improve matters give lignocaine 100 mg i.v. as a bolus and start an i.v. lignocaine drip to

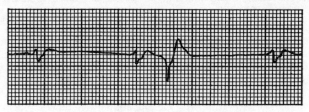

Fig. 10. *Ventricular ectopic beat.*

give 3 or 4 mg/min. Reduce this as soon as possible, usually within 1 hour, to the lowest level that suppresses the ectopic beats—usually 1 or 2 mg/min.

(2) If this fails, use:

    (i)   Disopyramide 50–100 mg i.v.[35]
    (ii)   Amiodarone 5–10 mg/kg i.v. over 1 minute then 600–1200 mg via a continuous infusion over 24 hours.

After myocardial infarction a few ventricular ectopics are very common—if they do not have the characteristics outlined in (1) (i)–(iv) above, just observe.

Ventricular tachycardia (Figs. 11 & 12)

(1) This may be difficult to distinguish from supraventricular tachycardia with bundle branch block because:

    (i)   The clinical signs which frequently occur in ventricular tachycardia namely:

        (a) occasional cannon waves,
        (b) varying intensity of first heart sound,

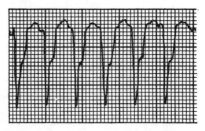

Fig. 11. There is no easily discernible P wave in this recording and it is impossible to tell whether this is supraventricular tachycardia with bundle branch block or ventricular tachycardia.

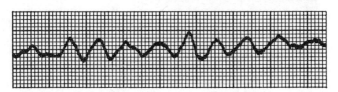

Fig. 12. *Ventricular fibrillation.*

are not always present and can occur in SVT with right bundle branch block.

and

(ii) The ECG features commonly associated with ventricular tachycardia namely:

(a) P waves in varying relationship to QRS complexes,
(b) slight irregularity of the QRS complex and rate may occur in either condition.

P waves are best seen in leads V1 and 2. They may be accentuated by a high V1 (i.e. in the interspace above the normal V1) by an S5 electrode (right arm electrode on the manubrium, left arm electrode on the fifth right interspace near the sternal edge, with the lead selection switch on S1) or by an oesophageal lead, or they may appear when the rate is slowed down by one of the drugs suggested below.

(2) Some help may be had from the forms of the QRS complex.

(i) If it is of right bundle branch form, then a triphasic complex, right axis deviation and an 'S' wave in V6 which is smaller than the 'r' wave are suggestive of SVT with aberrant conduction.

(ii) If it is of left bundle branch form, than a complex with negative deflection in V4 and V5 less than in V1, a normal or left axis and a narrow or absent 'r' wave in V1 are suggestive of SVT with aberrant conduction.

(iii) Ultimately, the origin can only be confirmed by electrophysiological studies.[31]

(3) Fortunately the treatment of choice for both ventricular and supraventricular tachycardia is synchronised reversion with a DC shock. Distinguishing between the two does not determine your immediate management.

(4) DC reversion is almost always effective. If it is not, check that the patient is not hypoxic, anxious or in pain or electrolytically unbalanced. If you do not have the equipment, or DC reversion is unsuccessful, use drugs as for ventricular ectopics. If the situation is deteriorating contact a specialist unit for advice. They may be able to offer either paired or coupled pacing.

(5) Digoxin should never be used in patients with ventricular arrhythmias.

(6) Following the correction of a ventricular arrhythmia, give lignocaine i.v. for 24 hours (*see* p. 15), in the expectation that this will prevent further episodes.

HEART BLOCK[33,34]

This is either:

(1) First degree which is defined as a P–R interval prolonged for more than 0·22 seconds (Fig. 13)—This occurs in digoxin overdosage, coronary artery disease, myocarditis and excessive vagal tone. It is of little significance and is not treated unless:

    (i)   it lengthens
           and/or
    (ii)   dropped beats start to occur.

Either may herald complete heart block and if (i) or (ii) occurs following a myocardial infarct, insertion of a temporary transvenous pacemaker should be considered.

(2) Second degree—Here the ventricles do not always respond to atrial contraction. There are two types of second degree block, first clearly distinguished by Mobitz, and designated Mobitz type I and type II.

    (i)   Mobitz type I—In this type of block, there is either a progressively lengthening P–R interval culminating in a dropped beat (the Wenckebach phenomenon (Fig. 14)) or the conducted beat has a prolonged P–R interval (Fig. 15a). The prognosis of Mobitz type I block is good and normal conduction may often be restored with atropine 0·6 mg i.v. or, failing this, dopamine (*see* p. 13). Only if these fail or the patient's cardiac output is compromised or the degree of block progresses should a pacemaker be inserted.

    (ii)   Mobitz type II—Here the conducted beat has a normal P–R interval (Fig. 15b). The ratio between non-conducted and conducted atrial contractions may be as great as 5:1. Mobitz type II block often progresses to complete heart block, and so here a transvenous pacemaker should be inserted as soon as possible. Sympatho-mimetic agents

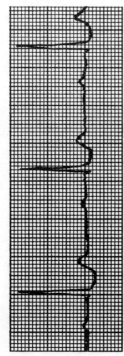

Fig. 13. *First degree heart block*. The P–R interval is greatly prolonged to 0·36 seconds.

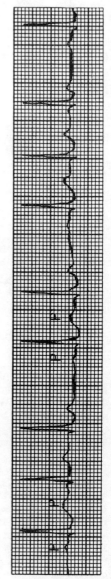

Fig. 14. *Second degree block. The Wenckebach phenomenon*. The first P–R interval of the sequence is prolonged. The second P–R interval is more prolonged and is seen deforming the preceding T wave. The third P wave is lost in the preceding T wave and the ventricle sometimes responds to this and sometimes fails to respond. Once the dropped beat has occurred the sequence is then repeated. (Mobitz type I block.)

28

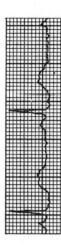

Fig. 15b. *Second degree block.* Normal P–R interval of conducted beat. (Mobitz type II block.)

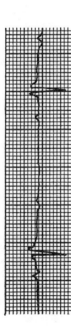

Fig. 15a. *Second degree block.* Prolonged P–R interval of conducted beat. (Mobitz type I block.)

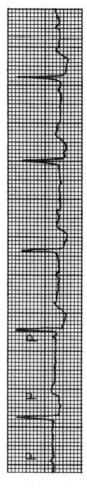

Fig. 16. *Complete heart block.* The first three P waves are marked. They can be seen to be beating quite independently of the QRS complexes.

29

should be used with care in this type of block, as an increase in atrial rate may increase the ratio of atrial to ventricular beats, and thus the ventricular rate may actually slow down.

(3) Complete heart block (Fig. 16)—Here the ventricular activity bears no temporal relationship to atrial activity. It is usually due to fibrous replacement of the conducting system, but may occur after myocardial infarction. It may rarely be caused by digoxin toxicity, or trauma to the bundle of His (e.g. after cardiac surgery).

Complete heart block may:

(i)   cause congestive cardiac failure,
(ii)   cause hypotension and poor tissue perfusion,
(iii) be punctuated by attacks of ventricular asystole, tachycardia or VF (Stokes Adams attacks).

Treatment

(1) Following myocardial infarction[29]—a temporary transvenous pacemaker should be inserted immediately, under fluoroscopic control.[32] Sinus rhythm usually returns within one week of infarction, but may take up to three. If it does not, permanent pacing will be required.

(2) In other circumstances—if the low heart rate is causing symptoms, a permanent pacemaker should be inserted, if necessary preceded by a temporary wire as in (1) above. If pacing is not available, or while things are being organised, either give i.v. dopamine (see p. 13) or alternatively 2 mg isoprenaline in 500 ml of dextrose, infused at a rate of 3–8 μg (10–30 drops/min), until the ventricular rate is above 60 beats/min.

(3) Complete heart block may be presaged by the following.

(i)   A lesser degree of block (see p. 27).
(ii)   A combination of left axis deviation (signifying left anterior hemi-block) and right bundle branch block (Fig. 17), or right axis deviation (signifying left posterior hemi-block) and right bundle branch block (Fig. 18). Both of these configurations imply that at least two out of three of the conducting bundles are damaged and some of these patients progress to a complete block.

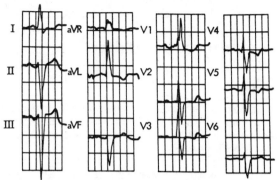

Fig. 17.   Right bundle branch block with left axis deviation.
By permission of Dr. D. O. Williams and Messrs Butterworth and Co.
(Publishers) Ltd.—publishers of Stock and Williams 'Diagnosis and
Treatment of Cardiac Arrhythmias'.

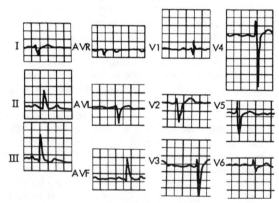

Fig. 18.   Right bundle branch block with right axis deviation.
By permission of Dr. D. O. Williams and Messrs Butterworth and Co.
(Publishers) Ltd.—publishers of Stock and Williams 'Diagnosis and
Treatment of Cardiac Arrhythmias'.

(iii)   The ECG configurations in (i) and (ii) above are an indication for pacing if:

(a) they develop after myocardial infarction;

(b) they are associated with symptoms attributable to
Stokes Adams attacks.

Acute pulmonary oedema

DIAGNOSIS

(1) Acute pulmonary oedema is usually caused by a rise in pulmonary capillary pressure overcoming the osmotic pressure of plasma proteins. This in turn is usually caused by left ventricular failure, in which case:

    (i) There is usually a history of increasing dyspnoea, fatigue, anorexia and orthopnoea which may be accompanied by a dry cough and possibly attacks of paroxysmal nocturnal dyspnoea with production of pink frothy sputum.

    (ii) Examination reveals a frightened, gasping patient who is pale and cyanosed with cold peripheries and who is pouring with sweat. The arterial pressure may be high with a narrow pulse pressure and in addition pulsus alternans may be present. A third heart sound and loud P2 may be present but are usually difficult to hear because of lung sounds—there are widespread loud crackles and wheezes over the lung fields. The sputum is pink and frothy.

    (iii) The chest x-ray is usually characteristic with semi-confluent mottling spreading from the hila, and enlarged upper lobe pulmonary veins. In addition there may be left ventricular enlargement, Kerley 'B' lines and pleural effusions, and the left ventricular end diastolic pressure will be raised—see (iv) and (v) below. There may also be evidence of an obvious cause.

    (iv) The Pulmonary Capillary Pressure (PCP) at which pulmonary oedema secondary to left ventricular failure occurs, depends on the serum albumin level. At a normal serum albumin level of 32 g/l, pulmonary oedema due to heart failure will only occur when the PCP is above 25 mmHg. At lower albumin concentration, pulmonary oedema will occur when the PCP is less than 18 mmHg. A simple formula (serum albumin (g/l) $\times$ 0·57 expressed as mmHg) gives a good approximation to this critical pressure.

    (v) The pulmonary capillary pressure is essentially the same as the left atrial pressure (which in its turn reflects the left ventricular end diastolic pressure). The left atrial pressure is usually measured indirectly using a Swan-Ganz catheter with its tip wedged in a small pulmonary artery (*see* p. 281).

(2) Pulmonary oedema can also occur in patients who are severely ill for other reasons (e.g. septicaemia, acute renal failure) and who do not have a raised left atrial pressure. Here the likely cause is transudation of fluid from damaged capillaries. The appearance and management of these patients differs from those in left ventricular failure (*see* section on shock lung p. 83).

(3) Acute pulmonary oedema has to be distinguished from:

(i) Asthma (*see* p. 69), for in both conditions the patient prefers sitting up, tachycardia is present, and both may have inverted T waves on the ECG. In asthma there is more high-pitched wheeze and fewer crackles than in acute pulmonary oedema. The patient is not grey and sweaty unless *in extremis* when parts of the lung fields are virtually silent; there is a quick inspiratory snatch and a prolonged expiratory phase; pulsus paradoxus may be present, the sputum is white and very sticky; the chest x-ray is usually normal or shows hyperinflation of the lungs. When, as sometimes happens, the main clinical evidence for pulmonary oedema is wheezing, the clinical situation and chest x-ray help distinguish it from asthma.

(ii) Pulmonary embolus (*see* p. 40).

(iii) Acute on chronic respiratory failure may mimic acute pulmonary oedema and be preceded by a history of orthopnoea. $Pa\text{co}_2$ before morphine and oxygen are given may help distinguish between the two, and must be measured if there is any doubt. Unfortunately, patients who have no pre-existing lung disease may sometimes have a raised $Pa\text{co}_2$ when in LVF.[42]

(iv) Other causes of acute shortness of breath (*see* p. 267) which are less easily confused.

(4) The causes of pulmonary oedema must be considered, especially the following treatable conditions.

(i) Myocardial infarction (*see* p. 8).

(ii) Severe hypertension (*see* p. 37).

(iii) Mitral stenosis and regurgitation, aortic stenosis and cardiac aneurysms.

(iv) Sub-acute bacterial endocarditis.

(v) Cardiac arrhythmias (*see* p. 17).

(vi) Water and salt overload, especially in an anuric patient.

(vii) Pulmonary embolus. This may so comprise oxygen supply to the heart, that left ventricular failure develops.

(viii) Cardiac tamponade.

(ix) Cardiomyopathy.

(x) Left atrial myxoma or ball valve thrombus (once in a lifetime).

MANAGEMENT

Management involves reducing the pulmonary oedema as follows:

(1) Sit the patient up if he has not already done so himself, either in a cardiac bed or with the legs over the side of the bed.

(2) Give:

(i) Oxygen by either MC mask or nasal catheter 4–6 l/min. If the patient has chronic respiratory failure give 24% O_2 initially by a Ventimask. If the Pao$_2$ is less than 40 mmHg increase the percentage of oxygen whilst monitoring the $PaCO_2$ (*see* p. 65).

(ii) Morphine 5–10 mg, and an antiemetic such as cyclizine 50 mg i.v. If the patient has chronic respiratory failure there is no safe sedation. If he is very distressed, probably the best thing to do is to give a small dose of morphine together with doxapram (1 mg/kg i.v.) and treat respiratory depression as necessary, whilst monitoring the blood gases.

(iii) Frusemide 40 mg i.v.

(iv) Aminophylline helps to reduce bronchospasm and in addition may lower the pulmonary venous pressure. A loading dose of 5 mg/kg slowly over 30 min followed by an infusion at 9 mg/kg/12 hour attains adequate blood levels safely, but may occasionally cause headache and nausea.

(v) A cardiac glycoside. If the patient has not had a cardiac glycoside within the last five days, give oubaine, a rapid-acting cardiac glycoside with a half-life of about 21 hours. The dose is 0·5 to 1·0 mg i.v. slowly repeated four-hourly as necessary to a maximum of 2·0 mg in 24 hours. The patient may later be transferred to digoxin (0·125–0·5 mg daily depending on size, age and renal function) for maintenance.

(3) Having given (ii)–(v) above, reassure the patient and then leave the nurse to make observations. Do not hover looking anxious. This will increase the patient's anxiety.

(4) If three-quarters of an hour later the patient is

    (i)   the same:

        (a) repeat the dose of lasix and
        (b) give a further 5 mg of morphine, both intravenously.

    (ii) worse:

        (a) let one pint of blood—this is best done with an ordinary blood donor's set
        (b) cuffing the limbs is now known to be ineffective in LVF.[43]

(5) If, despite these measures, the patient continues to deteriorate consider putting him on a ventilator. Positive pressure ventilation will reduce the venous return, lower the arterial pressure, and force the oedema back out of the alveoli. This may hold the situation until the other measures have taken effect.

Investigation and treatment of the cause

(1) A chest x-ray and ECG should be taken as soon as possible.

(2) If an arrhythmia is thought to be the cause, the ECG should be continuously displayed on an oscilloscope. The arrhythmia is treated in the usual way (see p. 17). In particular, atrial fibrillation may be an important contributory cause in an already jeopardised myocardium.

(3) Many patients with acute pulmonary oedema have a transiently elevated arterial pressure. However, if there is evidence of previous hypertension (hypertensive retinopathy, left ventricular hypertrophy) and the diastolic pressure is maintained at >110 mmHg steps should be taken to lower it (see p. 38).

(4) Acute pulmonary oedema in the following special circumstances:

(i)   Mitral stenosis—is an indication for an emergency valvotomy if the patient is already on adequate medical treatment.

(ii) Anuria—is an absolute indication for dialysis.

(iii) Papillary muscle and ventricular septa can rupture following myocardial infarction and may be amenable to surgical repair.

(iv) Cardiac tamponade—is an indication for paracentesis of the effusion without delay.

(v)   A cardiac aneurysm—intractable cardiac failure may be controlled by resection of the redundant muscle.

(vi) Atrial myxoma or ball valve thrombus—can be relieved, it is said, by re-positioning the patient, head down.

Hypertension[45]

DIAGNOSIS

(1) Hypertension may be regarded as an emergency when:

(i) It is causing left ventricular failure (*see* p. 32).

(ii) It is causing hypertensive encephalopathy. This causes periodic attacks of severe headache, accompanied by vomiting, convulsions, confusion, deterioration of vision, possibly focal neurological signs and eventually coma. On examination the systolic and diastolic arterial pressures are usually more than 200 mmHg and 140 mmHg respectively. The fundus shows florid hypertensive changes and the urine contains protein. Treatment is by reduction of the arterial pressure (*see* p. 38).

(iii) It occurs in association with dissections of an aortic aneurysm (*see* p. 49).

(iv) The diastolic arterial pressure is more than 140 mmHg.

(v) It occurs in association with acute or chronic renal failure (*see* p. 121).

(2) Three common pitfalls giving a high arterial pressure reading which do not in themselves require treatment are:

(i) A single arterial pressure reading taken shortly after first meeting a patient. The patient's outward calm may be belied by the accompanying tachycardia.

(ii) When the arterial pressure reading is artificially elevated by gross obesity.

(iii) When the systolic pressure is elevated by a rigid atheromatous aorta.

(3) The effect of a high arterial pressure can be seen directly in the fundus and can be inferred from clinical and ECG evidence, viz:

(i) Deepest S wave in right ventricular leads plus tallest R wave in left ventricular leads add up to more than 36 mm.

(ii) ST depression plus T wave inversion in left ventricular leads.

MANAGEMENT

Reduction of arterial pressure to a diastolic of 100 mmHg is all that should be attempted. Further reduction may reduce cerebral blood flow to such extent that neurological symptoms occur. Special care is needed in treating patients who have cerebral infarction with associated severe hypertension (*see* p. 169).

The arterial pressure may be lowered rapidly with any one of the following drugs:

(1) Sodium nitroprusside.[17, 49, 50] This is the drug of choice. If your pharmacy has no access to the ready made solutions, make up a fresh solution of 50 mg sodium nitroprusside in 500 ml of 5% dextrose (0·01% solution). This is given continuously i.v. An incremental infusion rate in the dose range 0·5–10·0 μg/kg/min should control the pressure, but doses up to 480 μg/kg/min have been used for short periods of time. It is mandatory to measure thiocyanate and cyanide levels with exceptionally high doses, but at doses of under 10 μg/kg/min no adverse side effects have been noted.[49] Cyanide poisoning can be reversed by giving hydroxy cyanocobalamin 1000 μg i.v. or, in severe cases, the specific antidote to cyanide poisoning, dicobalt EDTA in a dose of 300 mg i.v.

(2) Hydrallazine (Apresoline).[47] Give 10 mg i.m. or i.v. four-hourly as necessary. Common toxic effects are tachycardia, headaches, nausea and vomiting. Occasionally dizziness, flushing and sweating, dyspnoea, angina, paraesthesia and urticaria may occur.

(3) Diazoxide (Eudomid).[46] Give 5 mg/kg rapidly i.v. The dose may be repeated as necessary. Side effects are the development of hyperglycaemia and sodium and water retention.

Hydrallazine and diazoxide both increase cardiac stroke volume and cardiac work and in patients with dissecting aneurysm or with pulmonary oedema sodium nitroprusside or one of the following drugs is preferable.

(4) Ganglion blocking agents.

(i) Pentolinium tartrate (Ansolysen). Start with 2 mg subcutaneously. The effect lasts 45 minutes, and is best seen with the bed head elevated. Pentolinium should be given hourly until the desired effect is achieved, if necessary increasing the dosage each hour. Tolerance occurs over 10–12 weeks, and doses up to 100 mg/day have been given. The side effects are those of the ganglion blockers, i.e. postural hypotension, constipation, dryness of the mouth and difficulty with micturition. In addition some patients experience weakness, blurring of vision, diarrhoea, and occasionally may be nauseated at the start of treatment.

(ii) Trimetaphan. This has a short half-life, and acts immediately, so is given by i.v. infusion, the rate of which is adjusted in accordance with the arterial pressure response. The infusion dose is between 1 and 15 mg/min.

(5) Treatment with diuretics, in doses adequate to maintain urinary output, and oral hypotensives should start at the same time.

(6) Hypertensive crisis in phaeochromocytoma must be treated with an alpha adrenergic blocking drug. Give phentolamine 2·5–5·0 mg i.v. at five-minute intervals until the arterial pressure is controlled and thereafter at 2–4 hour intervals, or as needed to keep the arterial pressure under control.

Phentolamine may also be given as a continuous infusion at a rate of 0·2–0·5 mg/mm. Sodium nitroprusside may also be used in this situation.

Pulmonary embolus[50,59,60]

DIAGNOSIS

(1) Pulmonary embolus, depending on its size, may present as one of four clinical pictures, the last three of which may overlap to some extent.

Group A: Sudden death. The diagnosis is established at post mortem.

Group B: Acute dyspnoea which may or may not be accompanied by signs of shock (*see* p. 241). This needs to be distinguished from myocardial infarction (*see* below).

Group C: Pleuritic pain and haemoptysis, unaccompanied by signs of circulatory failure. This needs to be distinguished from pneumonia (*see* below).

Group D: Shortness of breath alone. This characteristically insiduous onset of multiple pulmonary emboli should always be considered in a patient with a history of slowly progressive dyspnoea.

(2) The signs on examination will again vary according to the size of the embolus:

(i) The signs of pulmonary hypertension may be present if approximately two-thirds of the area of the pulmonary arterial bed is obstructed. These signs, which occur in a major pulmonary embolus (Group B above), include:

(a) A giant 'a' wave in the jugular venous pulse.
(b) A powerful para-sternal heave.
(c) A right atrial gallop (triple heart sounds heard loudest in the pulmonary area).
(d) Accentuation of the pulmonary second sound.

(ii) The signs of pulmonary infarction. This does not invariably follow pulmonary embolus but is usually present if pleuritic pain occurs—characteristically Group C. A pleural friction rub is heard and if the infarct is large this is followed in about 48 hours by dullness, decreased breath sounds and crackles over the site of the infarct.

(3) The legs should always be examined for signs of deep vein thrombosis.[53] These thrombi, of course, are the source of the embolus.

The signs are:

(i) Delayed cooling of the exposed leg.
(ii) Increased size of the calf, the careful measurement of which should be compared with the other leg.

These are two of the most reliable signs of deep vein thrombosis.
In addition there may be:

(i) Accentuation of the venous pattern and oedema of the ankle and foot.
(ii) Tenderness on palpation of the calf muscles or Hunter's canal.
(iii) The presence of thrombi in the veins above the knee (the usual source of emboli) can be confirmed simply by ultrasound.
(iv) The absence of a DVT does not exclude a pulmonary embolus—all the clot may have travelled to the lung by the time of your investigations.

Remember that Homan's sign is falsely positive or falsely negative too often to be of any value, and that 70% of DVTs give rise to neither signs nor symptoms.

(4) Investigations include:

(i) Chest x-ray. Frequently there may be no evidence of large pulmonary emboli on any ordinary chest x-ray. Collapse of part of a lung may be inferred from an elevated diaphragm (the first sign to develop) and increased translucency of one lobe or lung. As the infarct becomes haemorrhagic the characteristic wedge shaped shadow appears. In addition, the pulmonary artery diameter may be enlarged (more than 17 mm in a man and more than 16 mm in a woman) or the pulmonary artery may even be seen to terminate abruptly—'pulmonary cut off'.
(ii) ECG. The ECG may be initially normal, but may change rapidly in the early phases of the illness. Characteristic patterns of change are:

(a) An attempt to develop right axis deviation—an S wave
     in I-a Q wave in III with a raised ST segment and
     inverted T wave (but not also in II as in inferior
     myocardial infarction) and inverted T waves across the
     right ventricular chest leads with clock-wise rotation
     (Fig. 19).

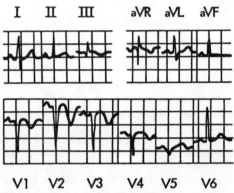

Fig. 19. ECG in pulmonary embolism. By permission of
Dr S. Oram from 'Clinical Heart Disease' published
by Heinemann Medical Publishers.

(b) Development of right bundle branch block.
(c) Any of the conventional ischaemic patterns, presum-
     ably provoked by low coronary artery blood flow.

(iii) A perfusion scan of the lungs may reveal areas of
       diminished flow at a time when the chest x-ray is normal.
       In a person with pre-existing lung disease it is helpful to
       combine the perfusion scan with a ventilation scan. A gross
       mis-match, showing under-perfusion of normally venti-
       lated areas, is characteristic of pulmonary embolism.
(iv)   Serum enzymes. Characteristically the lactic acid dehyd-
       rogenase is increased whilst the serum aspartate amino
       transferase (glutamic-oxaloacetic transaminase) is nor-
       mal. This combination helps to distinguish Group B from
       myocardial infarction. In addition, the serum bilirubin is
       raised (when the haemorrhagic infarct begins to break
       down) in about three-quarters of all patients with pulmonary
       emboli, and the patient may even be clinically jaundiced.

(v) Pulmonary arteriography is the only certain way of diagnosing pulmonary embolus. It may demonstrate absent or incomplete filling of the pulmonary vasculature. The indications for this investigation—which is quick and is of minimal inconvenience to the patient if the specialised equipment and experience is available—are discussed below. Retrograde venography undertaken at the same time may show the source of the embolus in the pelvic or leg veins.[52]

MANAGEMENT

Group A is fatal by definition. Group B is frequently fatal. Group C should always be treated urgently because some 30% of patients who survive one embolus have a second which is fatal in about 20%. Patients in Group D also require urgent treatment but are not, unlike Groups B and C, in mortal danger.

Management involves:

(1) Establishing the diagnosis. As indicated above, physical examination of the acute case may be helpful, but is seldom conclusive, and has to be considered together with the chest x-ray and ECG which should both be obtained as soon as possible. As already indicated pulmonary arteriography is the only certain diagnostic measure, and should be undertaken in any patient in whom there is clinical suspicion of a major pulmonary embolus. The radio-opaque dye used during arteriography is a vasodilator, and to prevent the possibility of a catastrophic fall in blood pressure during the examination, you should give phenylephrine 0·1–0·5 mg i.v. immediately prior to the examination.

(2) Restoring the systemic circulation. This is the first consideration in Group B and is most effectively achieved by moving the embolus.

How to do this is controversial, but:

(i) If the heart has stopped cardiac massage may not only restart it, but may also break up and disperse the embolus.

(ii) If the patient is in shock or deteriorating rapidly with signs of progressive right heart failure, pulmonary embolectomy should be undertaken. Heparin should then be used post-operatively. In less grave situations a trial of fibrinolytic therapy is justified.

(iii) Thrombolytics (fibrinolytics) may be infused into the pulmonary arteries through the catheter with which the arteriogram has been done.

Give either:

(a) Urokinase[54, 55] (which is expensive but not allergenic) 100 000–150 000 units/hour for 2 hours. If the initial response is unsatisfactory continue the infusion at the same rate to a total of 700 000 units, or

(b) Streptokinase[55, 58] (which is cheaper, but is allergenic). Give an initial dose of 500 000 units in 30 min and then infuse 100 000 units/hour for 72 hours.

Both these are hazardous, in that severe bleeding may occur during the infusion. This paradoxically may be treated by increasing the infusion rate (but consult the haematologists first).

(iv) Whilst definitive measures are being initiated, you may have to support the circulation. To this end, it is important to keep the right atrial pressure (and thus the right ventricular filling pressure) high. A pressure of 12 mmHg above the sternal angle appears to be optimal for maximising right sided stroke work in this situation. The right atrial pressure tends to be high anyway in major pulmonary emboli but if less than 12 mmHg infuse dextran 70 under CVP control. You will probably only need a few hundred cc, so be wary.

If raising the right ventricular filling pressure is to no avail, use inotropic agents (*see* p. 3).

(3) Reversing hypoxia, which is always present because intrapulmonary shunting, alveolar hypoventilation, and impaired perfusion occur. Oxygen via an MC mask is partly effective in relieving this hypoxia.

(4) Relieving pain. Give heroin (*see* p. 8).

(5) In Groups C and D the systemic circulation is not jeopardised and none of the measures (i)–(iii) is required. However, in all groups, whatever the initial treatment, further emboli can be prevented by anticoagulants. This should be undertaken as indicated on page 14.

Removal or exclusion of any remaining deep vein thrombi. These have first to be identified either by retrograde phlebography at the same time as the pulmonary arteriogram, or by bilateral ascending femoral phlebography. After identification either direct surgical removal or proximal ligation of the affected vein can be undertaken, depending on the site of the thrombus. An alternative is to infuse fibrinolytic agents locally or systemically, in the doses given above.

(6) Pregnancy—In the particular circumstances of pulmonary embolism in pregnancy, anticoagulation should be commenced with heparin, as advocated on p. 14. Warfarin is best not used since it is teratogenic and is also associated with an increased incidence of ante-partum haemorrhage.[57]

Peripheral embolus[62]

DIAGNOSIS

(1) Obstruction of blood supply to an organ usually causes acute loss of function with or without pain. The diagnosis should be considered when this occurs, especially when there is an obvious source of embolus, e.g. recent myocardial infarction, atrial fibrillation, mitral stenosis, etc.

(2) Thus:

(i) *In the limbs*—the patient complains of coldness and/or pain. On examination the limb is pale and cold and the peripheral pulses are absent. The diagnosis therefore is usually fairly clear. However, it may be mimicked by a deep vein thrombosis which occurs in a leg with pre-existing obstructive arterial disease. Here also the leg is painful, pale and pulseless, but may be differentiated from infarction by the development of oedema. In addition an arterial embolus is experienced first as pain which passes into numbness.

(ii) *In the gut*—causes abdominal pain with vomiting and possibly the passage of blood per rectum. There may be signs of peritonitis and impending intestinal obstruction. The patient rapidly deteriorates if infarction of bowel has occurred. Diagnosis is made at laparotomy.

(iii) *In the kidney*—the patient complains of acute loin pain and haematuria, symptoms which may also be caused by a stone. An IVP and renogram should distinguish between these two, and an arterial occlusion can be confirmed by selective renal arteriography.

(iv) *In the carotid circulation*—causes the onset of neurological signs, e.g. hemiplegia. If this occurs in a setting where an embolus is likely, early arteriography should be undertaken to determine the site of the block.

(3) Emboli are not infrequently multiple. All the peripheral pulses should be carefully palpated.

MANAGEMENT

Involves:

(1) *Eliminating the source of the embolus.* If possible this should be undertaken before the peripheral embolus is removed. If mitral stenosis is present the appendage of the left atrium should be secured and flushed out and mitral valvotomy performed whenever possible.

(2) *Removal of the embolus.* As a general principle this should be undertaken whenever possible. Thus:

   (i) *In the limbs*—surgery should be undertaken without delay, preferably after arteriography. The embolus may be removed under local anaesthetic. Therefore, the general condition of the patient is irrelevant, and a 'wait and see' policy is unjustified. Whilst the theatre is being prepared do not:

   (a) elevate the leg, causing decreased perfusion;
   (b) wrap up the leg, precipitating gangrene;
   (c) warm the leg, increasing metabolism;
   (d) cool the leg, causing vasoconstriction.

   If embolectomy is either unsuccessful or impossible, the following regimes may be helpful:

   (a) Alternate bottles of 20 ml 95% alcohol in 500 ml of saline with 500 ml dextran 70[61] in 5% dextrose six-hourly.
   (b) Thrombolytic therapy (in doses as for pulmonary embolism) has been attended by successful dissolution of clot (*see* p. 44).

   In this condition adrenergic blocking agents are valueless.

   (ii) *In the gut*—if at all possible, embolectomy and revascularisation of the bowel should be undertaken immediately. If infarction has occurred survival without operation is extremely rare.

   (iii) *In the kidney*—operation should be considered, at which either the embolus or the kidney is removed depending on the viability of the latter.

   (iv) *In the extra-cranial carotid arteries*—immediate embolectomy under local anaesthetic may be considered.

    (v)   *In the intra-cranial carotid*—anticoagulants should be started if the embolus originates from an extra-cranial source and the neurological deficit has resolved (*see* p. 173).

(3) *Prevention of further emboli.* If the primary thrombus cannot be reached a course of anticoagulants should be started (*see* p. 14) as they have been shown to reduce the incidence of further thrombi.

Dissections of the aorta

DIAGNOSIS

(1) The process of dissection may be intensely painful. Pain may be experienced in the chest, the back, the abdomen or the legs, depending upon the origin of the aneurysm and may spread from one site to another depending on the direction and extent of the dissection. In almost half the cases, however, pain is slight and the diagnosis is made from a chance finding on chest x-ray, from a sudden drop in the arterial pressure, or from the signs of ischaemia (*see* p. 46).

(2) The signs include the following.

    (i) Shock (*see* p. 241) which may be due to severe pain or to loss of blood.

    (ii) Signs of ischaemia in the:

        (a) myocardium—myocardial infarction;

        (b) limbs—apart from gross signs (*see* p. 46) a difference of 20 mmHg between the systolic arterial pressures of opposite limbs indicates arterial obstruction in the limb with the lower pressure;

        (c) brain—a hemi or quadriplegia;

        (d) kidneys—if both kidneys are involved, as is usually the case, there is severe oliguria with a few red cells or complete anuria;

        (e) gut (*see* p. 46);

        (f) spinal cord—paraplegia.

    (iii) Aortic regurgitation.

    (iv) Haemopericardium.

(3) Investigations include:

    (i) Chest x-ray. This should be repeated every 24 hours in order to detect changes in the contour of the aorta.

    (ii) Echocardiography. This may show widening of the aorta and the characteristic double lumen of the aorta. It can't be used to exclude dissection but may provide useful positive information.

(iii) Aortography. This is the definitive investigation for a dissecting aortic aneurysm and must be undertaken if operative treatment is considered.

MANAGEMENT

The priorities of medical management in order are as follows.

(1) Relief of pain. Any one of the following combinations may be given and repeated as often as necessary provided the patient is not dangerously hypotensive:

    (i)   Heroin 5–10 mg i.v. plus prochlorperazine 12·5 mg i.v.
    (ii)   Morphine 15 mg i.v. plus prochlorperazine 12·5 mg i.v.

(2) Lowering the blood pressure if raised (*see* p. 38).
(3) Relief of cardiac tamponade (*see* p. 51).

Further management should be discussed with a cardiovascular surgeon who should be consulted as soon as the diagnosis has been considered.

Cardiac tamponade

This term implies restriction of cardiac function by mechanical constriction of the heart. This is usually caused by a tense pericardial effusion, or by a haemopericardium (which may follow a dissecting aneurysm, a chest injury or a myocardial infarction). It may also be caused by blood clots surrounding the heart even when the pericardium has been left widely open, as after thoracic surgery.

DIAGNOSIS

(1) There may be a preceding history of precordial pain followed by increasing dyspnoea.

(2) The signs are those of:

   (i) *Decreased cardiac output.* Despite a tachycardia the patient is hypotensive, the pulse pressure is small and the peripheries are poorly perfused. In addition pulsus paradoxus is usually present. This may be demonstrated by measuring the systolic arterial pressure in expiration and inspiration. If there is a fall of >10 mmHg on inspiration then constriction is present.

   (ii) *Increased pressure in the systemic and pulmonary veins.* The jugular venous pressure is raised. The 'y' descent is rapid and there is a conspicuous 'y' trough. In addition the jugular venous pressure rises on inspiration.

   Similarly the respiratory rate is raised and the patient is occasionally orthopnoeic, with wheezes and possibly crackles in the chest.

   (iii) *The effusion itself.* It may be possible to demonstrate an increased area of dullness around the precordium. In addition, the apex beat is impalpable and the heart sounds are muffled. However, a third heart sound can usually be heard. Thus, the diagnosis should always be considered in a patient with severe left ventricular failure and/or hypotension.

(3) On screening, the cardiac outline is relatively immobile. The extent of the effusion may be estimated by cardiac catheterisa-

tion and angiography, echocardiography, or by a 'heart' scan with a radioisotope (technetium) tagged to the patient's red cells. The echocardiogram is the most reliable technique, and has the great advantage of being non-invasive.

(4) The ECG may be of low voltage and there may be widespread inversion of T waves.

(5) If cardiac tamponade needs to be relieved urgently, the signs are usually gross—the pulse almost disappearing on inspiration. This degree of severity may be caused by a surprisingly small effusion.

MANAGEMENT

(1) The heart must be decompressed:

    (i)   if the patient is distressed;

    (ii)   the systolic arterial pressure is <90 mmHg and/or the jugular venous pressure is more than 10 cm.

(2) (i)   If the patient is *in extremis* insert a wide bore needle in the fourth intercostal space over the precordium and advance until fluid is obtained. This may release enough fluid—often surprisingly little—to relieve the heart.

    (ii)   Otherwise the site of choice is the xiphisternal angle. Sit the patient up at 45°, insert the needle 3 cm below the xiphisternum at an angle of between 30° and 45° to the skin. Apply suction to the needle, and push it slowly upwards and backwards until fluid is obtained, and then aspirate as much fluid as you can. The heart may be difficult to feel, but usually produces ectopic beats when scratched. If you have your needle connected to an ECG machine, as you should, you will get an appropriate reading (Fig. 20).

    (iii) If the effusion is haemorrhagic, you may wonder if you have unwittingly entered a cardiac chamber. Place a few cc of the fluid in a glass tube—intracardiac blood will clot, haemorrhagic effusion will not.

    (iv) To minimise the chances of your entering a cardiac chamber, it is helpful to attach your aspiration needle to the 'V' lead terminal on the ECG cable. This can be done by means of an insulated wire with a clip on each end—

failing this, just attach the wire with Sellotape. Figure 20 shows the electrocardiograms obtained when the needle tip is advanced to three different sites.

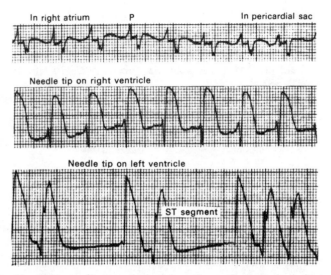

Fig. 20. Electrocardiogram obtained from the needle tip at three sites. Reproduced with kind permission of Dr. A. Hollman and the editors of 'Medicine'.

SECTION I REFERENCES

Cardiac arrest

1 Campbell NP, Webb SW, Adgey AA, *et al*. Transthoracic ventricular defibrillation in adults. *Br Med J* 1977; **2**: 1379.
2 Chamberlain DR. Cardiac arrest. *Br J Hosp Med* 1972; **8**: 251.
3 Goldberg AH. Cardiopulmonary arrest. *N Engl J Med* 1974; **290**: 381.
4 Kravitz AE, Killip T. Cardiopulmonary resuscitation: status report. *N Engl J Med* 1972; **286**: 1000.
5 Chandras N, Rudiboff M, Weisfeldt MI. Simultaneous chest compression and ventilation at high airway pressure during cardiopulmonary resuscitation. *Lancet* 1980; **1**: 175.

Myocardial infarction

6 Bradley RA. *Studies in acute heart failure*. London: Edward Arnold 1977.
7 Braunwald E. Reduction of myocardial infarction size. *N Engl J Med* 1974; **291**: 525.
8 Braunwald E. Coronary spasm and acute myocardial infarction. *N Engl J Med* 1978; **299**: 1271.
9 Chalmers RJ, Smith H Jr, Kunzler AM. Evidence favouring the use of anticoagulants in the hospital phase of acute myocardial infarction. *N Engl J Med* 1977; **297**: 1091.
10 Leader. Nitroprusside in myocardial infarction. *N Engl J Med* 1982; **306**: 1168.
11 Muller JE, Stone PH, Braunwald E. Let's not let the genie escape from the bottle again. *N Engl J Med* 1981; **304**: 1294.
12 Epstein SE, Kent KM, Goldstein RE, *et al*. Reduction of ischaemic injury by nitroglycerin during acute myocardial infarction. *N Engl J Med* 1975; **292**: 29.
13 Forrester JS, Diamond G. Chaterjee K, *et al*. Medical therapy of acute myocardial infarction by application of haemodynamic subsets. *N Engl J Med* 1976; **295**: 1356.
14 Hillis LD, Braunwald E. Myocardial ischaemia. *N Engl J Med* 1977; **296**: 971, 1034, 1093.
15 Leader. Hypotensive treatment for acute myocardial infarction. *Br Med J* 1975; **1**: 353.
16 Leader. Intravenous dopamine. *Lancet* 1977; **2**: 231.

17 Leader. Controlled intravascular sodium nitroprusside treatment. *Lancet* 1978; **2**: 784.
18 Leader. Surgery for coronary artery disease. *Br Med J* 1978; **1**: 597.
19 Multicentre trial by European working party. Streptokinase in acute myocardial infarction. *Br Med J* 1971; **3**: 325.
20 Sullivan JM. Streptokinase and myocardial infarction. *N Engl J Med* 1979; **301**: 836.
21 Warlow C, Terry G, Kenmore AC, *et al*. Double blind trial of low doses of subcutaneous heparin in the prevention of deep vein thrombosis after myocardial infarction. *Lancet* 1973; **2**: 934.
22 Webb SW, Adgey AA, Pantridge JF. Autonomic disturbance at onset of acute myocardial infarction. *Br Med J* 1972; **3**: 89.

Pre-infarction syndrome

23 Leader. Unstable angina. *Lancet* 1982; **2**: 569.
24 Leader. Calcium blocker therapy for unstable angina pectoris. *N Engl J Med* 1982; **306**: 926.
25 Leader. Coronary bypass surgery. *Lancet* 1973; **1**: 1937.
26 Sobel BE. Propranolol in threatened myocardial infarction. *N Engl J Med* 1979; **300**: 191.

Arrhythmias

General

27 Schamroth L. *The disorders of cardiac rhythm*. Oxford: Blackwell Scientific Publications, 1971.
28 Leader. Clinical implications of the diving response. *Lancet*; **1**: 1403.
29 Atkins SJ, Blomqvist G, Mullins CB. Ventricular conduction block and sudden death in acute myocardial infarction. *N Engl J Med* 1974; **288**: 281.
30 Atkinson JA. Diphenylhydantoin as an anti-arrhythmic drug. *Ann Rev Med* 1974; **25**: 99.
31 Kastor JA, Horowitz LN, Harken AH. Clinical electrophysiology of ventricular tachycardia. *N Engl J Med* 1981; **304**: 1004.
32 Harris AM. Transvenous pacing. *Br J Hosp Med* 1969; **2**: 1131.
33 Kastor JA. Atrioventricular block. *N Engl J Med* 1975; **462**: 572.
34 Kastor JA. Hemiblocks + stopped hearts. *N Engl J Med* 1978; **299**: 249.

35   Koch-Weser J. Disopyramide. *N Engl J Med* 1979; **300**: 957.
36   Lie KI, Wellens HJ, van Capelle FT, *et al.* Lidocaine in the prevention of primary ventricular fibrillation. *N Engl J Med* 1974; **291**: 1324.
37   Leader. Sick sinus syndrome. *Br Med J* 1977; **1**: 4.
38   Leader. Antidysrhythmic treatment in acute myocardial infarction. *Lancet* 1979; **1**: 193.
39   Leader. New approaches to antiarrhythmic therapy. *N Engl J Med* 1981; **304**: 475.
40   Singh BN, Hauswirth O. Comparative mechanism of action of antiarrhythmic drugs. *Am Heart J* 1974; **87**: 367.

Pulmonary oedema

41   Rosenbaum MB. Clinical efficiency of amiodarone as an antiarrhythmic agent. *Am J Cardiol* 1976; **38**: 934.
42   Leader. Blood gas tensions in acute pulmonary oedema. *Lancet* 1972; **1**: 1106.
43   Leader. Rotating tourniquets for left ventricular failure. *Lancet* 1975; **1**: 154.

Hypertension

44   Leader. Hypertensive encephalopathy. *Br Med J* 1979; **2**: 1378.
45   Koch-Weser J. Hypertensive emergencies. *N Engl J Med* 1974; **290**: 211.
46   Koch-Weser J. Diazoxide. *N Engl J Med* 1976; **294**: 1271.
47   Koch-Weser J. Hydrallazine. *N Engl J Med* 1976; **295**: 320.
48   Leader. Hypertensive encephalopathy. *Br Med J* 1979; **2**: 1387.
49   Palmer RF, Lasseter KC. Sodium nitroprusside. *N Engl J Med* 1975; **292**: 294.

Thrombo-embolism and pulmonary embolism

50   Adelstein JS. A new diagnostic tool for pulmonary embolus. How good and how costly? *N Engl J Med* 1978; **299**: 305.
51   Deykin D. Regulation of heparin therapy. *N Engl J Med* 1972; **287**: 355.
52   Dow JD. Retrograde phlebography in major PE. *Lancet* 1973; **2**: 407.
53   Deep vein thrombosis (symposium). Incidence; medical treatment; surgical therapy. *Br J Hosp Med* 1971; **6**.

54 Edwards IR. Low dose urokinase in major PE. *Lancet* 1973; **2**: 409.
55 Fratantoni JC, Ness P, Simon TL. Thrombolytic therapy: current status. *N Engl J Med* 1975; **293**: 1073.
56 Leader. Low dose heparin and the prevention of thromboembolic disease. *Br Med J* 1975; **3**: 447.
57 Leader. Thrombo-embolism in pregnancy. *Br Med J* 1979; 1661.
58 Leader. Streptokinase. *Br Med J* 1977; **1**: 927.
59 Miller JAH. Diagnosis and management of massive pulmonary embolus. *Br J Surg* 1972; **59**: 837.
60 Oakley CM. Diagnosis of pulmonary embolism. *Br Med J* 1970; **2**: 773.

Peripheral embolus

61 Perrson AV, Thomson J, Patman R. Streptokinase as an adjunct to arterial surgery. *Arch Surg* 1973; **107**: 779.
62 Thompson JE. Acute peripheral arterial occlusion. *N Eng J Med* 1974; **290**: 950.

RESPIRATORY

Respiratory failure[1]

DIAGNOSIS

(1) This is defined in terms of altered blood gases viz. an arterial oxygen tension (Pao_2) of less than 60 mmHg or an arterial CO_2 tension ($Paco_2$) or above 50 mmHg.

(2) Both hypoxia (low Pao_2) and hypercarbia (raised $Paco_2$) are difficult to pick up clinically because:

    (i) The classical signs of hypoxia are either non-specific (disturbances of consciousness, ranging from mild confusion to coma), or difficult to assess (cyanosis).

    (ii) Hypercarbia may give rise to a spectrum of mental changes similar to those of hypoxia. It may also cause a flapping tremor, peripheral vasodilation, papilloedema and early morning headaches, which again are not specific for a rising $Paco_2$.

Hence arterial blood gas measurements are mandatory if the diagnosis is suspected.

There are three patterns for respiratory failure:

(A) *Pure ventilatory failure* which gives rise to a raised $Paco_2$ and a low Pao_2. Examples of this are:

    (i) Depression of the respiratory centre by drugs.

    (ii) Neurological conditions such as poliomyelitis, myasthenia gravis, Guillain-Barré syndrome.

    (iii) Primary alveolar hypoventilation (Pickwickian syndrome).

(B) *Hypoxaemic failure* due to local disturbances of the ventilation perfusion relationship. This gives rise to a low Pao_2 with a low or normal $Paco_2$.[2] Examples of this are:

    (i) 'Pure' emphysema.

    (ii) Asthma in the initial stages of an attack (*see* diagram on p. 70).

    (iii) Pneumonia (*see* p. 86).

(iv) Left ventricular failure (but *see* p. 32).
(v)   Fibrosing alveolitis.
(vi) Shock lung (*see* p. 83).

(C) *A mixture of ventilatory and hypoxaemic failure*. This combination of alveolar hypoventilation and deranged ventilation perfusion relationships produces a low Pao$_2$ with a raised Paco$_2$. The example of this type of failure is chronic bronchitis with emphysema. Such patients frequently have a permanently low Pao$_2$ and may have a permanently high Paco$_2$ (and therefore a high serum HCO_3). Overt respiratory failure is usually precipitated by an acute infection with associated sputum retention, increasing airways obstruction and often heart failure. This is the commonest clinical setting for respiratory failure and the management of this is therefore discussed first.

ACUTE ON CHRONIC BRONCHITIS PRECIPITATING RESPIRATORY FAILURE

The patient often has a history of increasing breathlessness, increasing volumes of purulent sputum, and, occasionally, pleuritic pain. All this in the setting of chronic obstructive airways disease. Examination reveals a breathless, often pyrexial patient, who may be confused, cyanosed and have a tachycardia. There may be evidence of hypercapnia (*see* (2) (ii) above). There will be a prolonged expiratory phase, with variable crepitations and wheezes. The signs of collapse, consolidation, effusion or pneumothorax must also be sought, as any of these can exacerbate the situation. Signs of right sided heart failure (raised neck veins, oedema and a palpable liver) are often present.

MANAGEMENT

Initial investigations, in order of priority, are:

(1) Arterial blood gases and pH.
(2) Chest x-ray.
(3) Culture of sputum.
(4) Knowledge of haemoglobin, electrolytes and urea, whilst not often immediately useful, will be required.

The aim of management is to increase intracellular O_2. Experience with tissue oxygen electrodes is limited and as yet this is usually measured indirectly by the Pao$_2$. The Pao$_2$ should be increased to at least 45 mmHg and preferably to 50–55 mmHg, achieved preferably with a fall, or at least without a substantial rise, in the Paco$_2$.

Each of the factors enumerated in (C) above which contribute to the failure must be tackled.

(1) *Infection*. The commonest infecting organisms are *Strep. pneumoniae* and *H. influenza*. Both are usually sensitive to ampicillin 500 mg six-hourly (parenterally or orally), tetracycline 500 mg six-hourly (i.m. or orally, not i.v.) or co-trimoxazole tabs. ii b.d.

If the infection has been contracted in hospital, or if for other reasons you suspect that the infection may be caused by resistant staphylococci, add i.v. or i.m. cloxacillin 500 mg six-hourly.

If the sputum purulence has not decreased after 48 hours, consider changing the antibiotic, but consult your bacteriologist first. Remember that sputum culture and sensitivity tests may be misleading, so do not change antibiotics exclusively on the basis of information from these.

(2) *Sputum retention*. A patient's outlook may be transformed if energetic and regular physiotherapy 'raises the sputum'. Initially physiotherapy must be given two-hourly throughout the 24 hours, and if necessary you must teach both day and night nurses how to give appropriate physiotherapy. The sputum should be loosened by clapping the chest for 3–4 minutes, after which the patient should take a few quick deep breaths and then cough. Ideally this should be done in appropriate bronchial drainage positions. This is rarely feasible, but at least place the patient first on one side and then on the other. If the patient is too confused to co-operate, give physiotherapy after nikethamide. The sputum may be sticky, and intermittent humidification through a Wright's nebuliser can aid expectoration (4 ml of warm water is as effective as anything and is certainly cheapest).

If despite these measures the patient still cannot bring up sputum, it must be sucked up by either:

(i) Nasotracheal suction. Sit the patient up and with a gloved hand pass a soft catheter with a rounded end (off suction lest the pharynx and trachea be traumatised) through a nostril and into the pharynx. A convenient arrangement for this is to attach the catheter to one limb of a Y connector, which is itself attached to a sucker. Suction is then applied by occluding the other limb. To be of maximum benefit, the catheter must pass between the cords. Encourage the patient to cough, and as he exhales, advance the catheter and then suck.

If the patient cannot phonate, you are probably through the cords. Advance the catheter into each main bronchus in turn. This is a potent stimulus to coughing and you should leave the catheter down until no more sputum is forthcoming. If laryngospasm occurs, attempts to pass the catheter into the trachea should not be repeated.

(ii) Bronchoscopy. This should be undertaken if despite nasotracheal suction, the patient continues to deteriorate. Flexible bronchoscopes have made this a much less traumatic event than previously and, given the circumstances, the patient's memory for the event is hazy.

(iii) Tracheal toilet through an endotracheal tube.

(3) *Airways obstruction*. The reversible component may be due to:

(i) sputum retention,
(ii) mucosal inflammation,
(iii) bronchospasm.

Treatment of (i) and (ii) have been discussed. Bronchospasm must be assumed to be present, therefore:

(a) give salbutamol by nebuliser (10 ml salbutamol which is contained in 2 ml of nebulised salbutamol respirator solution) with intermittent positive pressure respiration over 3 minutes up to four times each day. Or failing this, by a pressurised aerosol (2–4 puffs every 4 hours);

(b) i.v. aminophylline 5 mg/kg initially and then 0·5–0·9 mg/kg/hour thereafter. As well as being a bronchodilator, aminophylline increases the force of diaphragmatic contraction, an important factor in this group of patients.[5]

(c) steroids may also be given (e.g. hydrocortisone 200 mg four-hourly) although the efficacy of these is arguable.

(4) *Oxygen therapy*.[4] Oxygen should be given in sufficient concen-

tration to raise the Pao_2 to at least 40 mmHg and preferably 55 mmHg. To aim higher than this is unnecessary and in view of the potential danger of oxygen therapy in this type of ventilatory failure, undesirable.

The danger of oxygen therapy arises because patients with a chronically raised $Paco_2$ rely not only on a rise in $Paco_2$ as normal, but on a fall in Pao_2 to stimulate respiration—the so-called 'hypoxic drive'. A sudden rise in Pao_2 may reduce this hypoxic drive, and thus depress ventilation. This causes a further rise in $Paco_2$ and may precipitate CO_2 narcosis.

So after you have measured arterial blood gases, start with the 24% oxygen mask.

Measure the arterial gases again after one hour.

If:

(i) The Pao_2 is above 55 mmHg and $Paco_2$ has not gone up by more than 10 mmHg continue using 24%.

(ii) The Pao_2 is below 55 mmHg and the $Paco_2$ has not gone up more than 10 mmHg progress to 28% O_2 by Ventimask (4 l/min). Measure the $Paco_2$ again in a further hour and if situation (ii) still obtains, you may progress to the 35% Ventimask (8 l/min).

(iii) The $Paco_2$ has risen more than 10 mmHg. You are in grave danger of inducing CO_2 narcosis. Do not increase (or lower) O_2 concentration but intensify all other aspects of treatment, particularly the conjunction of physiotherapy and respiratory stimulants. If the $Paco_2$ goes on rising, despite this, you will have to decide if intermittent positive pressure respiration (IPPR) should be used. This can be a difficult decision, and depends particularly on the usual respiratory status of your patient. If he is a respiratory cripple, then IPPR is unlikely to be of lasting benefit and you may have difficulty weaning him off the ventilator.

(iv) Occasionally, patients are given high oxygen concentration by mistake, or in ignorance. This may lead to the rapid development of CO_2 narcosis. It is always best to assume that deterioration in the condition of a patient with ventilatory and hypoxaemic failure is due to CO_2 narcosis. Faced with this deteriorating situation:

(a) do not immediately increase the inspired O_2 concentration;

(b) prevent anybody else from doing so;

(c) measure the blood gases;

(d) if the chest signs have changed, repeat the chest x-ray to exclude pneumothorax or massive pulmonary collapse;

(e) intensify physiotherapy;

(f) if the Pao$_2$ is above 55 mmHg and the Pao$_2$ either above 90 mmHg, or has risen by more than 10 mmHg from your initial reading, reduce the O$_2$ to 24% by Ventimask, and use a respiratory stimulant;

(g) if the Pao$_2$ is below 35 mmHg as well as Paco$_2$ being high, give a respiratory stimulant without altering the oxygen concentration until the Paco$_2$ has improved;

(h) keep measuring the blood gases. You may have to consider IPPR if things go on deteriorating.

(5) *Respiratory stimulants*. These are used to:

(i) wake up the patient and help him to co-operate;

(ii) counteract CO$_2$ narcosis (as above);

(iii) counteract respiratory depression.

Remember in this context, that you must not sedate patients in respiratory failure. In fact, always write NO NIGHT SEDATION on their charts, so that no one else sedates them either!

The best drug to use is nikethamide 2–5 ml i.v. repeated half-hourly as necessary.

Ethamivan 5% 2·5 ml i.v. may also be used, as may doxapram, in a dose of 1·5 mg/min, increasing by 0·5 mg/min at half-hourly intervals if there has been no improvement to a maximum of 3·0 mg/min.

If respiratory depression is due to opiates, naloxone, which is a specific opiate antagonist, can be used in doses of 0·4 mg given i.v. over 3 minutes. This may be repeated to a total dose of 1·2 mg.

(6) *Heart failure*. The measures outlined above result in a substantial diuresia. However, in the presence of gross or persistent CCF give:

(i) Diuretics.

(ii) Digoxin, particularly if the patient has uncontrolled atrial fibrillation. Patients in respiratory failure have an enhanced sensitivity to digoxin, which is therefore best not used unless there is atrial fibrillation.

(iii) Do not forget that weight is a useful indicator of fluid balance—so weigh your patient daily.

(iv) In polycythaemic patients, diuresis may cause increased sludging of blood, and precipitate thrombosis. This may be prevented by venesection of four units of blood, and replacement with an equal amount of dextran mol wt 40 000 (dextran 40). This in itself, may be sufficient to improve renal blood flow and initiate a diuresis.

PURE VENTILATORY FAILURE

(1) There are occasions when the underlying problem is rapidly reversible, i.e. administration of naloxone to persons with opiate induced respiratory depression (*see* above).

(2) If no such specific therapy is available, the initial decision is when to institute artificial respiration.

(3) To make a decision you have to make appropriate measurements:

(i) Minute volume (measured with a Wright spirometer). If this is over 4 l/min the patient is very unlikely to require artificial ventilation.

(ii) Vital capacity (measured with a portable, bedside vitalograph). If the vital capacity remains above 1·5 l artificial ventilation will probably be unnecessary. The vital capacity should be measured at least daily in patients with progressive neurological lesions.

(iii) The blood gases should be measured if there is any doubt about the patient's respiratory status. If the Paco$_2$ is raised, artificial ventilation should be instituted.

(iv) Physiotherapy should be given routinely to help prevent sputum retention and infection.

(v) In unconscious patients without a gag reflex, or patients whose disease affects swallowing as well as breathing, inhalation of secretion or vomit must be prevented, by passing an endotracheal tube.

(iv) All this should be done in conjunction with the anaesthetists.

HYPOXAEMIC FAILURE

Treatment of the underlying disease should of course be initiated.

(1) Oxygen may be given by an MC mask (which delivers a concentration of 50–60% to the mouth, if the flow rate is 6 l/min) as there is no risk of CO_2 narcosis. However, be sure not to raise the Pao_2 too high (above 100 mmHg) because high oxygen concentration can be damaging to lung tissue.

(2) Artificial ventilation is rarely necessary and need only be resorted to if the Pao_2 cannot be maintained above about 50 mmHg.

Severe attacks of asthma[10,15]

DIAGNOSIS

(1) Recurrent reversible attacks of wheezing are the hallmarks of asthma and if despite treatment such an attack lasts for more than 6 hours, this is a serious situation with a real risk of unexpected death.

(2) Pulmonary oedema may cause wheezing and mimic asthma quite closely (see p. 33) but other causes of dyspnoea (see p. 267) are usually easily differentiated from asthma.

(3) An attack is usually precipitated by a combination of factors, which include infection, allergy and emotion.

(4) Severe attacks are characterised by:

  (i)   The patient who is too breathless to speak.
  (ii) Tachycardia of more than 130 beats/min.
  (iii) Pulsus paradoxus.[7, 8, 13] In acute asthmatic attacks paradox is usually, but not invariably present. When it is present the degree of paradox reflects the degree of airways obstruction. In a severe attack the difference in systolic arterial pressure between inspiration and expiration may be as much as 100 mmHg, the normal difference being not more than 5 mmHg.
  (iv) A 'silent' chest. There is insufficient air being moved to cause a wheeze.
  (v)   Cyanosis.
  (vi) Hypercapnia. The diagram (Fig. 21) demonstrates that in most cases of asthma, the Paco$_2$ is low, and that a patient with a high Paco$_2$ is mortally ill. Some authorities suggest that any asthmatic who has a Paco$_2$ above 50 mmHg when first seen should be ventilated forthwith, but in most circumstances it is reasonable to undertake management as outlined below.

MANAGEMENT

Measurements of pulse rate, respiratory rate, degree of paradox and arterial blood gases are mandatory. So is an initial chest x-ray as a

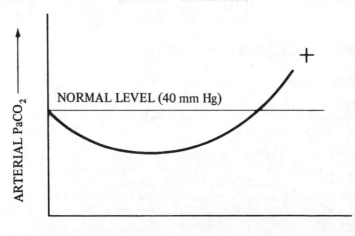

INCREASING SEVERITY OF ASTHMATIC ATTACK

Fig. 21.   Relationship between the Pa_{CO_2} and the severity of the asthmatic attack.

pneumothorax (*see* p. 73) or massive pulmonary collapse (*see* p. 76) may complicate an asthmatic attack, and require treatment in their own right. Peak expiratory flow rate (PEFR) and, if you have a spirometer, forced expiratory volume in one second (FEV1) are essential base-line measurements, changes of which provide a simple way of assessing progress.

Put up a drip and then treat:

(1) *The wheezing*.

   (i)   Hydrocortisone 300 mg i.v. stat. and 200 mg i.v. four-hourly thereafter until the patient is better.[7] Oral prednisone 40 mg/day should be started at the same time, as corticosteroids may take 6–8 hours to take effect.

  (ii) Aminophylline should be given at a loading dose of 5 mg/kg infused over 60 minutes, and 0·5–0·9 mg/kg each hour thereafter, aiming to obtain a serum level between 8–20 mg/l.[10]

 (iii) Adrenaline and isoprenaline should be avoided unless you can be *certain* that your patient has not been using an aerosol, in which case give adrenaline 1:1 000 0·5 ml subcutaneously.

(iv) Salbutamol. This is best given as an aerosol via a respirator; 2 ml of 0·5% salbutamol respirator solution contains 10 mg of salbutamol, and may be given up to four-hourly. Salbutamol may also be given intravenously, starting at a dose of 5 μg/min and increasing to 20 μg/min as necessary.

(v) Ipratropium bromide, an inhaled atropine-like compound causes bronchodilation by blocking vagal reflexes, and has a synergistic effect with salbutamol. Give 250 μg in 4 ml of solution by nebuliser on two occasions, 1 hour apart.[12]

(2) *Hypoxia*. Start by giving 28% O_2 via a Ventimask until you know the blood gases. If the Paco_2 is raised indicating that the patient's condition is critical, give O_2 as suggested on page 65, but bear in mind that ventilatory support will almost certainly be required in this group of patients. If the Paco_2 is below 40 mmHg, you can give any concentration of oxygen necessary to raise the Pao_2 to 80 mmHg.

(3) *Distress*. A severe asthmatic attack is alarming for all. However, you must not resort to sedation to allay the anxiety of your patient; rely on massive and repeated verbal reassurance. Try and exude confidence (which you will be far from feeling). Your patient's distress is entirely justified and he will be relieved as soon as he begins to get better and if he deteriorates, hypnotics only make matters worse.

(4) *Infection*. Recent trials have questioned the routine use of antibiotics in acute asthma. However, we feel their use is usually justified, so give either amoxycillin (250 mg i.v. six-hourly) or oral tetracycline (500 mg q.d.s.) or cotrimaxazole (tabs ii b.d.).

(5) *Dehydration*. Should be assumed to be present and should be corrected with adequate i.v. solutions (1·5 l of 5% dextrose and 500 ml of 0·9N saline in the first 24 hours is a reasonable amount, although up to six litres of fluid may be needed). Correction of dehydration helps make the sputum less tenacious.

(6) *Allergy*. Removing the patient to hospital often removes him from the allergen. Clearly you will use your observation in keeping him away from any allergens to which he has a known sensitivity.

(7) *Acidosis*. Correction with appropriate amounts of $NaHCO_3$ as calculated from the base deficit (*see* p. 245) can give rise to a considerable improvement.

(8) *Potassium*. Hypokalaemia often occurs in acute asthma, and potassium supplements should be added to the i.v. solutions as necessary.

(9) *Inspissated plugs of sputum*. These are present in the airways of most severe asthmatics. Physiotherapy is not likely to shift them, and is both impracticable and undesirable in the acute attack. As mentioned in (5) above, hydration is helpful in shifting these plugs.

(10) If your patient's clinical condition and arterial blood gases deteriorate despite the above measures, then ventilation with a powerful volume cycled respirator (IPPV) may well be necessary. In our experience, ventilation is rarely necessary, and only some 0·3% of patients in status require this support. It is important to have a drip up, preferably with a CVP line, before IPPV is instituted, as hypovolaemia may be unmasked by IPPV. Take the arterial pressure, pulse and CVP at 10-minute intervals and increase the infusion rate if necessary. This should be carried out in conjunction with your anaesthetic colleagues, and may be combined with bronchial lavage (*see* below).

(11) *Bronchial lavage*. Like ventilation this is only rarely required. It is carried out as follows (preferably by the anaesthetist!): the patient is intubated after injection of thiopentone followed by a muscle relaxant in the usual way. Inflate the lungs with 100% oxygen and ether. When the third plane of anaesthesia is reached, stop inflating and pour 1% sodium bicarbonate into the endotracheal tube until it overflows. Manually inflate three to four times and then perform endobronchial suction. Repeat this three or four times supine, in the left lateral, right lateral and Trendelenburg positions. This procedure, if properly carried out, may be effective in removing plugs of tenacious sputum, but carries the added risk of disseminating infection and causing further collapse. Then establish the patient on a volume cycled respirator at 12 to 15 cycles a minute and with a tidal volume of between 400 and 500 ml, observing the precautions in (10) above.

Pneumothorax[16,17,18]

DIAGNOSIS

(1) In a fit person:

    (i) Symptoms may be confined to slight dyspnoea or pleural pain, even when one lung is wholly collapsed.

    (ii) The signs are in combination diagnostic:

        (a) decreased movement on the affected side (not always present);

        (b) displacement of the trachea and apex beat (indicating mediastinal shift) may be present or absent, depending on the pressure in the pneumothorax;

        (c) increased resonance on the affected side (not always easy to detect);

        (d) distant breath sounds on the affected side (a good sign);

        (e) sometimes additional and often bizarre sounds may be heard—clicks or rubs;

        (f) the coin sign is rarely elicited but when it is, implies that the air in the pneumothorax is under increased pressure.

(2) However, the history, symptoms and signs may be absent, or be thought to have alternative explanation in patients who have other lung disease, such as emphysema or asthma. These patients may already be familiar from their previous episodes of infection or reversible airways obstruction— which look exactly similar. Their breath sounds may be difficult to hear at the best of times and a small pneumothorax may be impossible to detect. As they have no respiratory reserve and a missed diagnosis may be disastrous, they must always have a chest x-ray at each presentation.

(3) The association with Marfan's syndrome should not be forgotten.

(4) The diagnosis must be confirmed by a chest x-ray in expiration.

MANAGEMENT

Involves deciding:

(1) *When to insert an intercostal tube*. The indications are:

    (i)   if causing severe distress

        (a) In a fit person this means a tension pneumothorax which can cause cardiovascular collapse. The tension is relieved by letting air out of the chest. If the patient is *in extremis* insert a needle through the second inter-costal space in the mid-clavicular line. After the initial rush of air attach a syringe to the needle and insert an intercostal tube as soon as possible.

        (b) In a patient with co-existent lung disease where there is little or no respiratory reserve. As the hazards of pneumothorax are much greater in this group of patients it is probably wise to insert an intercostal tube even if severe dyspnoea is not yet present.

    (ii)   the presence of, or history of a pneumothorax on the other side

    (iii) if the lung is more than two-thirds collapsed.

(2) *The management of the tube*. The site of choice for insertion of the intercostal tube is in the mid-axillary line in the fourth or fifth intercostal space. The mid clavicular line in the second inter-costal space is poor alternative because sucking chest wounds have been known to occur after withdrawal of tube and it leaves an unsightly scar. The tube is attached to an underwater seal, e.g. a thoracotomy drainage bottle with 100 ml of sterile water in it, and the tip is directed up to the apex. Check the position on chest x-ray. Make the patient cough a few times every hour to allow the air to escape from the chest. If the level in the underwater tube stops swinging, either:

    (i)   The tube is blocked and it needs 'milking'. If this doesn't unblock the tube try and suck the tube free with a 50 ml syringe. If this doesn't work flush the tube out by introducing 50 ml of sterile water into the chest. Finally, change the tube.

    (ii)   The holes in the tube may be occluded by chest wall or partially re-expanded lung. Withdraw slightly and rotate.

(iii) The lung has re-expanded and is blocking off the end of the tube. In this case clip off the tube, re-x-ray 24 hours later and if the lung has gone down again continue to drain until the lung re-expands, then clip off, re-x-ray, etc.

(iv) If the lung does not expand even though the tube is patent, attach the outlet tube of the thoracotomy bottle to gentle suction (5–10 cm H_2O). Obviously the level will stop swinging. Take the tube off suction every hour to check that the tube is not blocked. If despite insertion of an intercostal tube and application of suction the lung still does not expand, consider bronchoscopy. This may clear the main airways of sputum and allow air to enter whilst the lung re-expands.

(v) If an air leak either persists or recurs:

    (a) check the connection of the intercostal tube to the drainage bottle;

    (b) seal the entry side of the intercostal tube in the chest by packing it with Tulle-gras to form an airtight dressing;

    (c) increase the suction pressure to 10–15 cm H_2O if the leak is very free. If the air leak continues there is probably a patent bleb on the lung surface. This will probably seal off in 36–48 hours. Keep the tube on suction until the leak stops. Suck for a further 12 hours, take off suction and watch the level in the underwater tube. If the chest maintains a negative pressure, i.e. the fluid level in the tube remains above the fluid level in the bottle, all is well. Clip off and re-x-ray in 24 hours. If the lung is still expanded take the tube out. If the two levels approximate and air begins to escape again, try sucking for a further 24 hours. If you are still unsuccessful pleurodesis should be considered and the advice of a thoracic surgical unit sought.

(3) Do not allow the thoracotomy bottle to be moved off the floor. If it is put on the bed locker, the contents will pass from the bottle into the chest. Keep two Spencer Wells clips on the thoracotomy bottle, and clip the tube off whenever you want to move the bottle or the patient.

(4) Physiotherapy—should be routine therapy for all patients with pneumothorax in an attempt to avoid sputum retention occurring. Remember to give any necessary pain relief prior to physiotherapy.[18]

Massive pulmonary collapse

Is the term used to express the complete collapse of a lobe or a lung. This may occur of course, due to a spontaneous pneumothorax or following a chest injury with a sucking chest wound. The following remarks are confined to the absorption collapse which follows occlusion of one of the main airways.

DIAGNOSIS

(1) May present itself as:

    (i)   sudden shortness of breath, with or without chest pain;
    (ii)   sudden worsening of an episode of acute infective bronchitis or asthma;
    (iii) fever, tachypnoea and tachycardia in an already ill patient, e.g. after major surgery;
    (iv) mental confusion.

(2) The signs are usually obvious. There is diminished movement on the affected side. The mediastinum is displaced towards the side of collapse as demonstrated by shifting of the trachea and apex beat. There is dullness to percussion. If the major bronchi are obstructed the breath sounds are diminished and there are usually no crackles. However, if the major bronchi remain patent but the peripheral bronchi are obstructed, the signs are those of consolidation, i.e. bronchial breathing, crackles and increased conduction of the spoken and whispered voice.

(3) Is most commonly caused by:

    (i)   a tenacious plug of sputum;
    (ii)   a foreign body which may be radio-opaque, e.g. classically a fragment of tooth after dental anaesthesia;
    (iii) carcinoma;
    (iv) extrinsic pressure on the bronchus, e.g. hilar glands, aortic, aneurysm, etc;
    (v)   occasionally, at intubation performed for any reason, the endotracheal tube may be inserted into one of the main bronchi, thus causing collapse of the other lung.

MANAGEMENT

(1) If the diagnosis is suspected a chest x-ray–PA and the appropriate lateral film should be taken. This will demonstrate the volume of lung collapsed; possibly also a foreign body in the trachea or bronchi or malposition of an endotracheal tube.

(2) Is directed towards removal of obstruction and obviously depends on the cause (*see* above). The two most common causes are:

    (i) *Sputum*. If the patient is severely hypoxaemic or comatose as, for example, after an operation, bronchoscopy should be undertaken immediately. Apart from this contingency there should be time to measure the blood gases. If the $Paco_2$ is raised it is probably advisable to proceed with bronchoscopy forthwith. If the $Paco_2$ is not raised it is permissible to delay 12 hours and await the effects of vigorous physiotherapy with chest percussion and coughing in the appropriate position. If at the end of that time there has been no improvement (as judged by a second chest x-ray) bronchoscopy should be undertaken.

    (ii) *Foreign body*. Removal through a bronchoscope should be undertaken without delay. Other causes are less common and, as they are not usually amenable to urgent treatment, are outside the scope of this book.

Acute laryngeal obstruction[20]

DIAGNOSIS

(1) Is usually obvious with severe distress coughing stridor, and enormous but ineffectual respiratory efforts. If not rapidly relieved, the victim may become blue, and then unconscious. In serious obstruction, speech is impossible.

(2) The cause is also usually fairly obvious:

    (i)   a foreign body which in adult practice is usually a piece of food inhaled while the victim is eating;

    (ii)   angio-neurotic oedema;

    (iii) severe burns;

    (iv) inhalation of irritant gases;

    (v)   trauma;

    (vi) carcinoma;

    (vii) after DXT to the neck;

    (viii) infections—classically diphtheria.

(3) Should not be confused with the obstruction caused by the tongue flopping back into the pharynx. This is of course easily relieved by lifting the jaw forward and inserting a pharyngeal airway.

MANAGEMENT

Involves:

(1) *Establishing a better airway*. This is indicated without delay if despite enormous respiratory efforts the patient is still cyanosed, and where the obstruction is due to an inhaled foreign body, is most expeditiously accomplished by using the Heimlich manoeuvre (*see* (3) below). It is also indicated (there being time to measure the blood gases) if hypoxia and CO_2 retention are present.

    (i)   In circumstances where the Heimlich manoeuvre is inappropriate or has failed, if there is time, spray the pharynx with a local anaesthetic (e.g. 5% cocaine and adrenaline). You will then be able to visualise the cords directly, and:

(a) determine the cause of obstruction—if this is not already apparent;
(b) remove a foreign body if one is present with a pair of long-handled forceps;
(c) pass an endotracheal tube.

(ii) If you do not have the necessary skill or equipment to pass an endotracheal tube, or if the obstruction is causing deformity of the larynx sufficient to make it impossible to pass an endotracheal tube between the cords (e.g. trauma, acute oedema) a tracheostomy must be performed. If the patient is *in extremis* this may be performed by a person with no surgical training. Pass a knife horizontally through the cricothyroid membrane and then twist the blunt end of the knife vertically to maintain the airway until a more formal tracheostomy can be established. An elective tracheostomy should be performed if the face is burnt, especially if there is evidence of burns inside the mouth or if the patient has a dry cough indicating tracheal involvement. This latter sign is also a useful warning if there is a history of inhalation of irritant gases.

(2) *Treatment of the cause.* Three types of obstruction may be rapidly relieved:

(i) foreign bodies, which must be removed as soon as possible preferably by employing the Heimlich manoeuvre;
(ii) angioneurotic oedema;
(iii) post radiotherapy oedema.

(ii) and (iii) may respond dramatically to hydrocortisone 200 mg i.v. Other forms of obstruction are usually treated after a tracheostomy has been performed and are not included within the scope of this book.

(3) *The Heimlich manoeuvre*[19]

(i) The principal here is that a rapid upward thrust from below the xiphisternum pushes the diaphragm up, and forcefully expels air from the mouth. Any obstructing object is likewise forcefully and dramatically expelled.

(ii) The technique can be carried out in people sitting, stand-
      ing or lying:

  (a) *Victim sitting or standing*. The rescuer either stands or
      kneels behind the victim, encircling the victim's waist
      with one of his arms. With one hand, he makes a fist,
      and places his thumb slightly above the navel, and well
      below the tip of the xiphoid process, then covers the fist
      with his free hand, and presses into the victim's abdo-
      men with a quick upward thrust. It may be necessary to
      repeat this thrust up to six times, although 60% of
      people are relieved of their obstruction after only two
      thrusts. The obstructing object may be expelled with
      such force as to hit a wall twelve feet away, and should
      be identified whenever possible.

  (b) *Lying victim*. Place the victim on his back, with his face
      looking directly forward. Facing the victim, the rescuer
      kneels astride him. He puts the palm of one hand
      between the navel and xiphisternum, places the other
      on top of it, and pushes upwards and inwards.

Massive pleural effusions[15]

DIAGNOSIS

(1) The patient usually has dyspnoea and may give a history of pleuritic pain.

(2) Differentiation from other causes of shortness of breath (*see* p. 267) is usually obvious on examination—the signs on the affected side being decreased movement, shift of the mediastinum to the opposite side, stony dullness, and decreased breath and voice sounds.

(3) The diagnosis is confirmed by a chest x-ray (*see* below).

MANAGEMENT

(1) The effusion must be aspirated if causing distress, whatever the cause.

(2) A chest x-ray–PA and the appropriate lateral—should be taken to determine the optimal site for aspiration and to delineate structures which must be avoided, such as the diaphragm. The diaphragm is attached to the sixth rib anteriorly, the seventh rib laterally and the ninth rib posteriorly. The sixth space laterally, or eighth space posteriorly (tip of the scapula) are recommended aspiration sites.

(3) If you do need to aspirate the effusion withdrawing fluid via a 50 ml syringe is tedious and prolongs discomfort for the patient. Therefore, insert a needle into the chest in the normal way. Attach it to the wall suction, if you have it, via a sterile underwater seal as for a pneumothorax (*see* p. 74) and by a gentle negative pressure (5–10 cm H_2O) aspirate fluid from the chest. If wall suction is not available; an evacuated sterile bottle can be used.[21]

(4) Stop aspirating if:

    (i)   a litre is obtained;

    (ii)   the patient complains of central chest pain. This means mediastinal shift is beginning to occur. This can cause rapid cardiovascular collapse and the temptation to continue must be resisted;

    (iii)   the patient has an haemoptysis. This means that the lung surface has been pierced. It is not usually serious but is frightening to all concerned. Unless the needle has been advanced further than necessary, the lung has re-expanded sufficiently for aspiration to be stopped.

(5) If the effusions are bilateral, aspiration of the larger effusion is usually sufficient to relieve dyspnoea.

Adult respiratory distress syndrome (shock lung)[22,24,26,28]

DIAGNOSIS

(1) Shock lung is characterised by:

    (i)   Tachypnoea;

    (ii) Deteriorating Pa_{O_2};

    (iii) Progressive diffuse infiltration on the chest x-ray occurring in a patient who within the preceding 48 hours has had an episode of hypotension.

(2) Is particularly likely to occur if the hypotensive episode was associated with:

    (i)   Traumatised or dead tissue, as in crush injuries;

    (ii) Circulating bacterial endotoxins, as in gram negative septicaemia;

    (iii) Fat emboli;

    (iv) Amniotic fluid emboli;

    (v) Intra-vascular haemolysis;

    (vi) Difficult or lengthy surgery.

(3) Arises because of an increase in:

    (i)   Pulmonary capillary permeability;

    (ii) Pulmonary vascular resistance.

    Both of these cause an increase in pulmonary interstitial fluid.

(4) Is associated with a normal pulmonary capillary wedge pressure (PCWP) initially. In shock lung PCWP will be below 18 mmHg and is most reliably measured using a Swan-Ganz catheter (*see* p. 281) wedged in the lower half of the lung field. By contrast in left ventricular failure, from which it must be distinguished, the PCWP is more than 25 mmHg, provided that the serum albumin is normal (*see* p. 32).

TREATMENT

Treatment is difficult, often prolonged, frequently unsuccessful and should be undertaken together with your anaesthetic colleagues. It involves:

(1) Therapy directed toward the specific insult provoking shock lung.
(2) Early assisted ventilation. You should attempt to keep the Pao_2 between 70 and 100 mmHg with added inspired oxygen, and introduction of positive end expiratory pressure (PEEP) of up to 10 cm H_2O. Remember PEEP may drop the blood pressure and this will be a limiting factor in its use.[29]

Indications for ventilation are:

   (i)   Respiratory rate of above 35/min.
   (ii) Pao_2 of less than 70 mmHg in spite of added O_2.[30]
   (iii) Alveolar arterial oxygen differences (A–aDO_2) of greater than 50.

The A–aDO_2 reflects the effective transfer of oxygen from the alveolus to the arterial blood. In a patient breathing room air with a Pao_2 of 150 mmHg.

$$A\text{–}aDO_2 = 150 - (Pao_2 + Paco_2)\ 0{\cdot}8$$

and is normally less than 20. (The value $0{\cdot}8$ in the above equation is the respiratory quotient.)

   (iv) Rising $Paco_2$. If the $Paco_2$ is above 40 mmHg, you have left things too late.

(3) Careful fluid balance

   (i) which fluids—

      (a) Blood should be replaced if the hematocrit falls below 30%.
      (b) High molecular weight dextran (dextran 70) should be used to expand the plasma volume if necessary (*see* below).
      (c) Crystalloid fluids should only be used sparingly to replace losses, as these fluids will of course tend to leak into the lung and aggravate the underlying problem.

(ii) How to monitor replacement. This is difficult because:

(a) If your patient is on a ventilator, and having PEEP, central venous pressure readings are unreliable.

(b) PCWP recordings only help to exclude co-existent left ventricular failure.

(c) Therefore, clinical judgement is of paramount importance. You should strive towards a patient with warm peripheries, good urinary output, clear mental faculties and an arterial pressure above 90 mmHg systolic, but, if in doubt, err on the side of keeping your patient 'dry' rather than 'wet'.

(4) *Antibiotics:* As infection does not seem to play an important role in the genesis of shock lung, only use antibiotics if there is purulent sputum.

(5) *Corticosteroids:* There is no evidence that these are helpful once shock lung has developed. Massive doses (2 g solumedrone i.v. each day for 2 days) may be helpful if inhalation of vomit has occurred.[27] If there is bronchospasm, hydrocortisone in the same doses as used for acute asthma (*see* p. 70) should be used.

(6) *Acidosis:* A low pH increases capillary leakage. Cautious correction with $NaHCO_3$ (*see* p. 246) with due regard to Na^+ balance, should be attempted.

(7) *Urea:* Likewise a raised urea (above 15 mmol/l) increases capillary leakage—careful attention to fluid balance and nutrition will help forestall this problem.

(8) *Cimetidine i.v.* should be given (*see* p. 114) as this lessens the tendency of very ill patients to develop, and bleed from, acute erosions.[19]

(9) *Physiotherapy:* Atelectasis occurs early in the shock lung syndrome. Encouraging regular sighing or deep respirations, making sure your patient coughs and is turned frequently, are vital therapeutic manoeuvres.

(10) *Membrane oxygenation:* Trials are underway to evaluate this novel, but as yet unproven, form of therapy.[23]

Fulminating pneumonia

Pneumonia is often the terminal illness in the elderly, and as such, should be managed on its merits. Fulminating pneumonia can, however, occur in otherwise healthy adults. It may strike with extraordinary rapidity, and at its most severe, someone who appears well in the morning may be dead by evening. The pathology of this condition is probably bacterial superinfection of a lung already damaged by a viral pneumonitis. The usual bacterial pathogen is staphylococcus, but *Strep. pneumoniae* and Klebsiella have been implicated. In some cases, a virus alone is thought to be responsible, frequently the influenza virus.

DIAGNOSIS

(1) There has often been a preceding viral illness, which may have seemed trivial. The symptoms are those of rapidly progressive dyspnoea, fever, cough productive of yellow and often bloodstained sputum and pleuritic pain. In the severest cases, there may be progression through mental confusion and disorientation to a state of septic shock with circulatory collapse. In these circumstances you may be presented with a hypoxic cyanosed disorientated, peripherally cool, hypotensive patient, and in this group mortality is high.

(2) The auscultatory signs are those of widespread, often asymmetrical areas of diminished breath sounds. There may also be focal evidence of consolidation, and an accompanying pleural rub. Chest x-ray usually shows non-specific diffuse lung shadowing.

MANAGEMENT

Take blood for arterial blood gases, FBP, including white cell count, electrolytes, and urea and blood cultures. Also, save a specimen for viral antibodies. Do a CXR and ECG and send sputum for Gram staining and culture. Then treat:

(1) *Hypoxia*. Profound hypoxia ($Pao_2 < 50$ mmHg) is the rule in this type of patient. Correction should be with 100% oxygen by MC

mask, whatever the initial $Paco_2$. If the Pao_2 persists below 60 mmHg or the $Paco_2$ persists above 40 mmHg on face mask oxygen, assisted ventilation will be required, and you should consult with your anaesthetic colleagues.

(2) *Infection.* Unless the Gram stain unequivocally demonstrates otherwise, it is best to assume you are dealing with the staphylococcus. Therefore give:

   (i) Penicillin—200 mg/kg per 24 hours as four-hourly doses i.v. together with flucloxacillin 500 mg i.v. six-hourly.
   (ii) Alternatively, if the patient is allergic to either of the above drugs give erythromycin 300 mg i.v. six-hourly and fucidin 500 mg i.v. six-hourly.
   (iii) If either of the above have been used without effect for 24 hours, or if at any stage your patient is desperately ill, it is reasonable to add metronidazole (*see* p. 249) and gentamicin (*see* p. 248).

(3) *Physiotherapy.* This is usually given to help your patient cough up infected sputum. Although its role in these circumstances has not been evaluated, we think it reasonable to give it.

(4) *Circulatory collapse.* In patients who develop circulatory collapse, the prognosis is very grave. Conventional therapy involving fluid replacement under CVP control (*see* p. 275) should be instituted. The only practical difference is that we suggest using predominantly colloid (plasma or dextran 70) rather than crystalloid to support the circulation. This is in an attempt to reduce the extravasation of fluid into the already damaged lung which will occur more readily with crystalloid. Insertion of a Swan-Ganz catheter, enabling you to measure pulmonary artery and pulmonary wedge pressure, will help you manage fluid replacement in these patients. Exudation of fluid into the lungs of these patients is usually due to parenchymal lung damage. This may be clinically difficult to distinguish from left ventricular failure, but by measuring the PCWP with the Swan-Ganz catheter, you should be able to distinguish between the two (*see* p. 9).

(5) *Steroids.* Their role is equivocal. However, on the grounds that solumedrone 2 g i.v. each 24 hours for 2 days may have some beneficial effect in septicaemic shock, we use steroids in patients who appear to be septicaemic.

(6) As always in these critically ill patients the care given by highly skilled nurses in an ITU is a critical factor in determining the outcome. You forget this at your patient's peril.

SECTION II REFERENCES

General

Crofton J, Douglas A. *Respiratory disease.* Oxford: Blackwell Scientific Publications (2nd Ed), 1975.
Hunter AR. *Essentials of artificial ventilation of the lungs.* London: Churchill Livingstone, 1972.

Respiratory failure

1 Clark TJH. Respiratory failure. *Br J Hosp Med* 1972; 7: 692.
2 Flenley DC. Clinical hypoxia—causes, consequences and correction. *Lancet* 1978; 1: 542.
3 Leitch AG. The hypoxic drive to breathing in man. *Lancet* 1981; 1: 428.
4 Woo SW, Hedley Whyte J. Oxygen therapy—the titration of a potentially dangerous drug. *Br J Hosp Med* 1973; 9: 487.

Asthma

5 Rochester DF. Is diaphragmatic contractility important? *N Engl J Med* 1981; 305: 278.
6 Fitchett DH, McNicol MW, Riordan JF. Intravenous salbutamol in the management of status asthmaticus. *Lancet* 1975; 1: 53.
7 Knowles GK, Clark TJH. Pulsus paradoxus as a valuable sign indicating severity of asthma. *Lancet* 1973; 2: 1386.
8 Knowles GK, Clark TJH. Pulsus paradoxus in asthma. *Lancet* 1978; 1: 940.
9 Leader. Corticosteroids in acute severe asthma. *Lancet* 1975; 2: 166.
10 Leader. Acute severe asthma. *Lancet* 1981; 1: 313.
11 Leader. Intravenous versus inhaled salbutamol. *Lancet* 1978; 1: 80.
12 Ward MJ, Fentem PH, Roderick Smith WH. Ipratroprium bromide in acute asthma. *Br Med J* 1981; 1: 598.
13 McGregor M. Pulsus paradoxus. *N Engl J Med* 1979; 301: 480.
14 Stark JF. Status asthmaticus. *Br J Hosp Med* 1972; 8: 241.

Spontaneous pneumothorax

15 Graham VA, Milton AF, Knowles GK. Routine antibiotics in hospital management of acute asthma. *Lancet* 1982; 418.

16 Kent Harrison G. Tension pneumothorax. *Br J Hosp Med* 1972; **8**: 246.
17 Leader. Spontaneous pneumothorax. *Br Med J* 1975; **2**: 526.
18 Crompton GK. Spontaneous pneumothorax. *Hospital Update* 1982, p. 251.

Acute laryngeal obstruction
19 Editorial. Statement on the Heimlich manoeuvre. *JAMA* 1975; **234**: 416.
20 Lockey RG. Allergic emergencies. *Med Clin Nth Am* 1974; **58**: 144.

Massive pleural effusion
21 Rutowska J. An easy method of aspiration for pleural effusions. *Hospital Medicine* 1967; **2**: 370.

Shock lung
22 Blaisdell FW, Schlobohm RM. The respiratory distress syndrome. *Surg* 1973; **74**: 251.
23 Leader. Membrane oxygenation in pulmonary failure. *Lancet* 1977; **2**: 390.
24 Leader. Pulmonary hypertension in acute respiratory failure. *Lancet* 1977; **2**: 283.
25 Leader. Gastro-intenstinal bleeding in acute respiratory failure. *Br Med J* 1978; **1**: 531.
26 Leader. Shock lung. *Lancet* 1977; **1**: 29.
27 Leader. White lipped anaesthesia (Mendelson's Syndrome). *Lancet* 1977; **2**: 123.
28 Pontoppidan H, Geffin B, Lowenstein E. Acute respiratory failure in the adult. *N Engl J Med* 1972; **287**: 690.
29 Cassidy SS, Gaffney AF, Johnson RL. A perspective on PEEP. *N Engl J Med* 1981; **304**: 421.
30 Leader. Acute oxygen therapy. *Lancet* 1981; **1**: 980.

GASTRO-INTESTINAL

Massive upper G.I. haemorrhage

(1) Presents itself as:

   (i)   Haematemesis and/or blood PR (melaena).
   (ii) Cardiovascular collapse.
   (iii) Postural hypotension and fainting.
   (iv) Symptoms of anaemia—fatigue, shortness of breath and angina, which however more often result from chronic blood loss.

(2) Is usually caused by:

   (i)   Bleeding peptic ulcers (possibly drug induced—*see* (ii) below).
   (ii) Acute gastric erosions.[11] These may:

         (a) be drug induced (salicylate, steroids, phenylbutazone and indomethacin being common offenders);[6]
         (b) occur after an alcoholic binge;
         (c) occur in any patient seriously ill for whatever reason.

   (iii) Reflux oesophagitis, with or without hiatus hernia.
   (iv) The Mallory-Weiss syndrome[4] (traumatic oesophageal tear usually secondary to prolonged retching or vomiting).
   (v)   Bleeding oesophageal or gastric varices (look for evidence of liver diseases).

(3) It may occasionally be caused by:

   (i)   gastric neoplasm;
   (ii) coagulation disorder (look for bleeding elsewhere, including prolonged bleeding from puncture sites);
   (iii) connective tissue disease, such as Osler-Weber-Rendu syndrome (look for telangiectasia).

MANAGEMENT

Management of this emergency always requires close collaboration between surgeons and physicians and sometimes radiologists, and every case should be treated jointly, preferably in an intensive care unit.

Management involves:

(1) **Restoration and maintenance of circulating volume and hence tissue perfusion.** This is urgent if blood loss sufficient to cause poor peripheral perfusion has already occurred (*see* p. 247) or the patient has a systolic arterial pressure of below 90 mmHg and a pulse rate of above 100 beats/min. It is always necessary to take cases of G.I. blood loss seriously as patients may continue to bleed in hospital. Therefore in all cases of major bleeding:

    (i)   Take blood for haemoglobin PCV electrolytes and urea, group and cross match 2 litres initially (and save the serum in case more blood becomes necessary) and kaolin cephalin time, prothrombin time and platelet count. But remember, haemoglobin concentration may be misleading before haemodilution occurs.

    (ii)   Set up a central venous pressure line.

    (iii) Replace the circulating volume. Two basic questions must be answered.

(A) *What with?*

    (a)   Compatible blood is clearly the fluid of choice, and should be available within a few hours.

    (b)   If the situation is not desperate, give 0·9% N saline whilst waiting. However, if you consider that a colloid is necessary before compatible blood is available, give:

    (c)   Plasma, or

    (d)   Dextran with an average molecular weight of 70 000 may be used; do not give doses in excess of 15 ml/kg/24 hour as they may cause disseminated intra-vascular coagulation. Dextran 40 is an alternative (*see* p. 243). Do not forget to take blood for cross matching before giving this.

    (e)   In desperate circumstances 'O' negative blood may be given uncross-matched.

(B) *How much?*

    (a)   If you have a CVP line (which you should have) transfuse blood rapidly until the CVP rises into the upper half of the normal range (i.e. 1 cm above the manubrio-sternal joint with the patient supine). The patient will become warm and tranquil and the arterial pressure and pulse will return to normal. If this does not happen, it implies the patient is continuing to bleed, and you must, therefore, continue to transfuse (whilst, of course, considering other possible therapeutic manoeuvres q.v.).

If after your initial resuscitation has been successful, the CVP drops suddenly (i.e. a fall of greater than 5 cm H_2O in less than 2 hours) this should be taken as an indication of re-bleeding. Further indications such as a fresh haematemesis or fresh blood up the naso-gastric tube, a fall in arterial pressure, or restlessness and sweating may then develop. All these will alert you to the need for further blood, and action (q.v.).

(b) If you have no CVP measurements, transfuse the patient until he is warm, tranquil and has a restored arterial pressure and pulse rate. A rate of about one pint of blood/hour is reasonable to start with.

(c) In all cases look for the usual clinical signs of overload (raised JVP, creps at the lung bases, oedema). If these occur slow down the infusion rate and give a diuretic, e.g. frusemide 40 mg i.v., and oubaine (*see* p. 34).

(iv) Consider passing a naso-gastric tube. This has the advantage that:

(a) it rids the stomach of Guinness, pills and blood;
(b) it may be useful in diagnosing re-bleeding;
(c) it may be helpful to know the pH of the stomach contents, so the appropriate dose of antacids or cimetidine can be given;
(d) the stomach can be emptied prior to endoscopy;

However:

(e) it is uncomfortable and sometimes is distressing for the patient;
(f) it may cause further bleeding;
(g) its use is associated with an increase in respiratory complications.

The authors do not use it routinely.

(v) In some patients, particularly the elderly who have had gradual blood loss, it is wise to give frusemide from the onset of the transfusion, as heart failure develops easily in this group.

(2) **Determining the cause.** This is undertaken when initial resuscitation is under way, and may be suggested by your history and examination.

Further investigations are:

(i)   Endoscopy, which we usually carry out within 24 hours of the patient's admission.[3, 5, 8] Although the site of bleeding will be visualised in most cases, giving comfort to physician and patient alike, early routine endoscopy has not altered the outlook in upper G.I. haemorrhage.[10] However, it is worth remembering that patients with liver disease may bleed from peptic ulcers as well as from varices, and actually seeing the bleeding site will sort this problem out for you.

(ii) If the patient continues to bleed rapidly after admission, the stomach is likely to be full of blood, and endoscopy unrewarding. In these circumstances arteriography gives a high degree of diagnostic accuracy, and is probably the investigation of choice.[17] It takes only half-an-hour and can be done whilst a theatre is being prepared, if the surgeons consider operation is necessary. Arteriography may also be an invaluable therapeutic technique (q.v.).

(iii) Emergency barium or gastro-grafin meals may be helpful in the diagnosis of upper G.I. bleeding (particularly where endoscopy is not available). You should consult with the radiologist as soon is practical.

(3) Stopping the bleeding

(A) *Peptic ulcer*

(i)   Cimetidine. A recent controlled trial showed no benefit from this drug so far as prevention of re-bleeding is concerned;[7]

(ii) Surgery undertaken to control bleeding may be considered if:

(a) the patient continues to bleed for 12 hours after admission;

(b) the bleeding recurs in hospital;

    (c) the patient is over 50;

    (d) there is a previous history of bleeding, or a long history of ulcer trouble;

    (e) if there is co-existence of another complication (e.g. perforation);

    (f) there is no more blood available.

(B) *Acute gastric erosions*[11]

    (i)   Surgery should be avoided if possible as the condition is usually self limiting.

    (ii)   Cimetidine—100 mg i.v./hour in 5% dextrose should be infused, with the aim of maintaining the pH of the stomach contents above 5.[2]

    (iii) Antacids—The best tested method of raising the pH of stomach contents is by instilling 30 ml of antacid (e.g. Maalox) hourly into the stomach. This may have advantages over cimetidine.[12]

(C) *Oesophageal or gastric varices*[12, 13, 14]

    (i)   Give vasopressin 20 units i.v. in 100 ml of 5% dextrose over 10 minutes. This substance lowers the portal venous pressure, and an effective dose causes pallor, colicky abdominal pain and evacuation of the bowel. It also causes coronary artery vasoconstriction, and should be used with caution in patients with ischaemic heart disease. The effect lasts about 45 minutes and the dose may be repeated four-hourly.

         If it is available, you should use the new analogue of vasopressin, triglycyl lysine vasopressin. This has a longer half-life than vasopressin, causes less side effects, and is more effective.[15] 2 mg are given by bolus intravenous injection six-hourly. If bleeding persists, this dose may be doubled.

    (ii)   If facilities for arteriography are available, the vasopressin is best given directly into the coeliac axis (at a dose of 0·2–0·7 units/min for 20 minutes).[1]

    (iii) If vasopressin fails, the Boyce modification of the Sengstaken Blakemore tube may be used.[16] A new tube should be used on each occasion, the upper G.I. tract should be aspirated via a naso-gastric tube, and the bed head should be elevated 6–10 inches. Then spray the pharynx with 2% lignocaine, test the balloons for leaks, make sure which tube connects with which balloon, and with the patient in a left lateral position pass the well-lubricated tube into the stomach. You may have to use a flexible wire to stiffen the tube if you have problems passing it. Fill the stomach balloon with about 100–150 cc of radio-opaque dye to localise it (20 ml of 20% diodone in 100 ml of water) and inflate the oesophageal balloon to a pressure of 30 mmHg. The oesophageal balloon must not be inflated until the tube has been stabilised by the stomach balloon. Similarly, the nursing staff must be told that they must always deflate the oesophageal balloon before emptying the stomach balloon, otherwise the oesophageal balloon may ride up the oesophagus and obstruct the pharynx. With the stomach tube pulled firmly up against the oesophago-gastric junction, tape it either to the patient or preferably, a preformed traction pad.[16]

Both during insertion and when the tube is finally in place, constant low pressure (5 mmHg) suction should be applied to the accessory tube, which aspirates secretions from the oesophagus and hypo-pharynx; this ensures that the oesophagus is kept free from potentially dangerous secretions. Both balloons are left in place for 24–48 hours, as necessary, then the oesophageal balloon deflated. The tube is left in position another 24 hours with the stomach balloon still full in case of re-bleeding. It is then removed (after emptying the stomach balloon!). No food or drink is allowed whilst the tube is in place, though drugs may be given via the stomach tube.

If used with care, the Sengstaken Blakemore tube will control oesophageal variceal bleeding in 90% of cases.[16]

The volumes of air and water mentioned above relate only to the Boyce modification of the Sengstaken tube, other varieties have different specifications and you should check this before using your tube.

(iv) In view of the ineffectiveness of any shunting or transection procedures to control bleeding, local injection of sclerosing agents into the varix (through a rigid or flexible gastroscope) is being tried—preliminary results are encouraging.[13]

(v)   Percutaneous trans-hepatic portal vein catheterisation, with subsequent selective injection of gel-foam into the major venous supply of the varices (left gastric and short gastric veins) is a promising new technique.[18]

(D) *Oesophageal bleeding due either to reflux oesophagitis or the Mallory-Weiss Syndrome*

(i) Medical measures usually suffice, but if bleeding persists surgery may become necessary.

(ii) Local arterial perfusion with vasopressin 0·2–0·4 i.u./minute for up to 36 hours may give temporary and sometimes permanent relief.

(4) **Arteriography as a therapeutic manoeuvre[1, 17]**

(i) This has already been mentioned in connection with oesophageal or gastric varices and tears.

(ii) In any other patients in whom torrential bleeding persists and in whom surgery is not desirable or possible one of two manoeuvres are helpful.

    (a) if the lesion is acute and superficial, or in the region of mesenteric perfusion, bleeding may be controlled by vasopressin 0·2–0·4 i.u./minute given for up to 36 hours.

    (b) if the lesion is chronic, arterial embolisation via the catheter is probably the treatment of choice.

(5) **General measures**

(i) The patient should be allowed to take fluids as required and offered a liberal soft nutritious diet with aludrox 10 ml every two hours. Both these help neutralise stomach contents.

(ii) Sedation should be given to an anxious patient. Restlessness, which is often a manifestation of hypoxia, may respond to oxygen and transfusion. Remember the potential danger of oxygen therapy before giving it (*see* p. 65).

(iii) Measure the urinary output, as renal failure may supervene on gastro-intestinal bleeding.

Ulcerative colitis[20,21]

Ulcerative colitis is characterised by widespread superficial ulceration of the colonic mucosa. It is a relapsing disease characterised by episodes of bloody diarrhoea. The severity of any single episode is related to the extent of colon involved, and, to a lesser degree, the severity of mucosal ulceration. In about 70% of episodes the colonic involvement is restricted to the sigmoid and rectum. Such cases do not usually constitute medical emergencies. However, more extensive involvement of the colon can give rise to a fulminant and potentially fatal disease. Appropriate management depends on accurate assessment of the severity of the attack.

DIAGNOSIS AND ASSESSMENT OF SEVERITY

(1) The diagnosis of ulcerative colitis is made by the association of:

   (i)   Clinical features (*see* below).
   (ii) *Sigmoidoscopic appearances*. The rectum is involved in 95% of all cases, and sigmoidoscope evidence of the disease will always be present in an acute attack. The mucosa will be uniformly oedematous and red, there will be multiple small ulcers or petechial haemorrhages, and free pus in the lumen of the bowel. The colonic mucosal wall will bleed on contact, and biopsy will provide histological evidence of the disease.

   Sigmoidoscopy *must* be carried out on all patients with a fresh attack of ulcerative colitis as it is the quickest and easiest way of substantiating the diagnosis.
   (iii) *Barium enema abnormalities*. In severe colitis, it is safe to perform a limited enema on an unprepared patient. Run in a small quantity of barium, remove it, and then insufflate a little air. This provides a good double contrast enema, and will help you diagnostically, as well as giving an indication of the extent and severity of colonic involvement.

(2) Features helpful in identifying a severe attack are:

   (i)   *More than six liquid, blood-stained stools in 24 hours—*

Patients with mild colitis frequently pass blood separately from faeces and it is the association of liquid faeces and blood which is important here.

(ii) *Fever*—A mean evening temperature of greater than 99·5°F.

(iii) *Tachycardia*—A mean pulse rate greater than 90 beats/min.

(iv) *Anaemia*—This is usually a combination of the anaemia of chronic disease and the anaemia of blood loss. Hb levels below 10·0 g/100 ml indicate serious disease.

(v) *An ESR above 30 mm/hour.*

(vi) *Hypo-albuminaemia*—Patients with ulcerative colitis may exude up to 30 g/day of protein through their raw colonic mucosa.

(vii) *Electrolyte disturbances*—Electrolyte and fluid loss through the inflamed mucosa may also be considerable, and hypokalaemia, hypocalcaemia and hypomagnesaemia all occur.

(viii) *Abdominal pain*—Pain prior to, and relieved by, defaecation is common in all grades of severity. Central abdominal pain, and colonic tenderness on palpation usually indicate a severe attack.

(ix) *Straight x-ray of the abdomen*—Dilation of the colon (>6 cm), mucosal islands, or gas under the diaphragm in a patient with severe colitis are all indications for immediate surgery.

(x) It should be noted that the systemic complications of ulcerative colitis (arthropathy, skin rashes, iritis and liver disease) do not necessarily relate to the severity of the bowel involvement.

DIFFERENTIAL DIAGNOSIS

Bloody diarrhoea and systemic disturbance may be a feature of:

(i) *Amoebic dysentery*. A history of foreign travel, characteristically foul smelling stools, the typical flask shaped ulcer on sigmoidoscopy and a positive amoebic complement fixation test will help you. Amoebae in the stools must be specifically looked for as they are easily confused with white cells.

(ii)   *Dysentery*. Usually caused by Gram-negative bacteria of the Shigella or para-typhoid groups. Send stool and a rectal biopsy specimen for cultures and enquire after contacts. This disease may produce rectal changes indistinguishable from ulcerative colitis on sigmoidoscopic examination.

(iii) *Crohns disease*. Classically Crohns involvement of the colon is patchy and the ulcers are deeper and serpigenous. However, as the management of acute Crohns colitis is essentially the same as that of acute ulcerative colitis, the differentiation of these two conditions is not an immediate priority.

(iv)   *Pseudomembranous colitis*. In this form of colitis, which characteristically occurs in an ill patient who has been given antibiotics, particularly clindamycin, yellowish adherent plaques are seen on sigmoidoscopy. The likely causal agent is *Clostridium difficile*, and the illness responds well to vancomycin 125 mg orally six-hourly.[19]

(v)   The rectal bleeding in ulcerative colitis is not usually severe. This, plus the characteristic sigmoidoscope findings, serve to distinguish it from several other conditions which may present with severe rectal bleeding, such as ischaemic colitis, diverticular disease, carcinoma of the colon and haemorrhoids.

MANAGEMENT

(1) Like most G.I. emergencies, management is best undertaken jointly by physicians and surgeons.

(2) Take blood for FBP and ESR serum Fe and folate, albumin and liver function tests, electrolytes including Ca^{++} and Mg^{++}, and urea. Do a daily, straight x-ray of the abdomen. Culture blood and stool.

(3) Correct the metabolic disturbances.

(i)   *The fluid disturbances*. Anorexia, pyrexia and enteric losses give rise to considerable fluid electrolyte and protein depletion. Initial replacement should be 0·9% N saline; preferably under CVP control. Hypoproteinaemia may be treated by colloid containing fluids, for example two units of plasma or its equivalent, each 24 hours.

(ii)   *Electrolytes*.

  (a) Na$^+$ deficiency is corrected as above.
  (b) Plasma K$^+$ is usually low. If less than 3·5 mmol/l give 3 g KCl (39 mmol) in each litre of replacement fluid. Otherwise re-measure 6 hours later and replenish as indicated.
  (c) If the plasma Ca^{++} is less than 2·3 mmol/l give 10 ml 10% calcium gluconate solution (2·25 mmol/day).
  (d) If the plasma Mg^{++} is below 1·0 mmol/l give 1 ml of 50% magnesium sulphate solution (2·0 mmol/day).

(iii) *The anaemia*. This is best corrected by blood transfusion. It is reasonable to aim at a haemoglobin level of 11·0 g/100 ml.

(iv)   *Nutrition*. Although there is no hard information on the subject most authorities suggest that patients with severe colitis should take non-milk containing fluids only. A convenient oral regime is 40 ml/hour of Vivonex dripped through a Clinifeed fine bore naso-gastric tube. If this is not possible i.v. feeding should be considered.

(4) *Suppressing the inflammation*. If there is no indication for immediate surgery (*see* below), give:

(i)   Prednisone 60 mg i.v./day. This is the drug of choice.
(ii)   *Antibiotics*. The role of bacteria in either initiating or exacerbating ulcerative colitis is unclear. Bacteraemia in association with severe ulcerative colitis is common, and some authorities advocate the routine use of metronidazole, penicillin and gentamicin (*see* pp. 248–9).
       Salazopyrine does not confer additional benefit in an acute attack and causes anorexia.

(5) *Surgery*. In most severe cases of colitis a trial of medical management is preferable. However, if the patient is not improving by 10 days, or, at any stage, deteriorates, total colectomy should be undertaken. The exact timing of such an operation has to be decided between physician and surgeon. However, immediate surgery is *always* required in the presence of:

(i)   *Toxic dilation of the colon*. This diagnosis is suspected when prostration accompanies a distended and tympanitic abdomen and is confirmed by a straight x-ray of the abdomen. The widest diameter of the colon should be less than 6 cm. Toxic dilation occurs only when virtually the entire epithelium of the colon has been destroyed. Mucosal islands or pieces of stripped off epithelium may hang from the colonic wall and be visible on the straight x-ray. This mucosal island sign is a further important pointer to immediate surgery.

(ii) *Perforation*. Colonic perforation may not cause specific symptoms or signs but is associated with a general clinical deterioration. The diagnosis is confirmed by the presence of air under the diaphragm on an upright abdominal x-ray.

(iii) *Profuse haemorrhage*. This is, however, extremely uncommon even in severe colitis.

(6) It is worth stressing again that treatment of this disease requires combined medical and surgical approach. Initial treatment with prednisone neither precludes nor complicates later surgery.

Medical conditions which may present with acute abdominal pain[22]

DIAGNOSIS

Abdominal pain may arise from stretching, violent contraction, ischaemia or infarction of the viscera, or from muscle, skin, bone, blood vessels, and nerves overlying or adjacent to the abdomen. It is not, therefore, surprising that many medical conditions can give rise to abdominal pain, and cause diagnostic confusion with an acute 'surgical' abdomen. In any patient presenting with abdominal pain, a careful history and a pause for reflection whilst necessary investigations are being performed and, where indicated, a trial of medical therapy is undertaken, may make an occasional laparotomy unnecessary. The following group of conditions should be considered.

(1) **Intrathoracic causes**

As the lower six thoracic nerves supply both thorax and abdominal wall, and as the heart and pericardium rest on the diaphragm, thoracic problems often cause abdominal pain—usually in the upper abdomen.

Important causes are:

(i) myocardial infarction (*see* p. 8);
(ii) pericarditis;
(iii) pulmonary embolus (*see* p. 40);
(iv) pleurisy;

all of which have characteristic clinical, radiographic, and ECG findings.

(2) **Intra-abdominal and retroperitoneal causes**

(i) *Acute pancreatitis*, which is often associated with gall stones, and sometimes with alcohol, hypercalcaemia, hyperlipidaemia and mumps. Take a plain x-ray of the abdomen, and look for the sentinel loop or pancreatic calcification. Do a serum amylase, blood calcium and look for methaemalbumen.

(ii)   *Congestion of the liver*, occurring in congestive cardiac failure and acute hepatitis, both of which should be looked for.

(iii)   *Acute pyelonephritis*, this typically causes loin pain and frequency, but sometimes the pain may be confined to the bladder area. Examine a fresh m.s.u. under the microscope and send some for culture.

(iv)   *Bowel ischaemia*, which may be due to:

    (a)   *Sickle cell diseases*. This should be considered in any one of African extraction with a history of jaundice. The patient may have parietal bossing and a characteristic facies.

    (b)   *Henoch-Schonlein purpura*. Abdominal pain may occur before the other signs, such as joint pains, rash haematuria and rectal bleeding, appear.

    (c)   The vasculitic lesions of polyarteritis nodosa, systemic lupus erythematosis, and other allied conditions may give rise to bowel pain. Given the clinical setting, the diagnosis is usually obvious.

(v)   *Constipation*. This can, of itself, cause severe abdominal pain, especially in the elderly. Rectal examination and a straight x-ray of the abdomen will reveal all.

(vi)   *Infection*,

    (a)   Gastro-enteritis causes colic, usually in association with diarrhoea and vomiting. A careful history will help you here.

    (b)   *Worms*. Tape worms can cause quite severe abdominal pain. Ovae and cysts should be looked for in the stools if a history of infestation is elicited.

    (c)   *Primary peritonitis*. This is an uncommon condition, usually occurring in patients with ascites. It is particularly liable to occur in children with the nephrotic syndrome. Aspiration of the abdominal fluid may reveal a cloudy aspirate from which diplococci may be grown.

(3) Metabolic and endocrine causes

(i)   *Diabetes*. You will diagnose this by finding glucose and ketones in the urine and a raised blood glucose. Of course, appendicitis can precipitate diabetic coma. However, it is reasonable to see if treatment of the diabetes relieves the pain within four hours or so, before proceeding to laparotomy.

(ii) *Hypercalcaemia*. There may be a history of constipation polyuria, polydipsia, renal calculi and mood disturbance. Look for the typical deposits of calcium at the corneoscleral junction.

(iii) *Porphyria* (usually of the acute intermittent variety). The urine contains increased quantities of prophobilinogen which is oxidised to porphobilin—a brownish coloured substance—when the urine is allowed to stand for half an hour.

(iv) *Addison's disease*. This may also cause vomiting, hypotension and peripheral circulatory collapse (*see* p. 151). The patient may have the characteristic pigmentation, and the diagnosis is confirmed by measuring the plasma cortisol.

(v) *Heavy metal poisoning—Classically lead* (look for the blue line on the gums—blood and urine lead levels and urinary coproporphyrins I and III are increased). Antimony, and cadmium may also cause abdominal pain.

(4) Neurogenic causes

(i) Compression of nerve roots by either malignancy or local degenerative lesions. The pain is usually band-like, and may give rise to segmental hyperaesthesia over the abdomen.

(ii) *Tabes dorsalis*. Attacks of vomiting associated with severe epigastric pain and lasting for several days may occur in tabes dorsalis. The presence of irregular pupils reactive to accommodation but not to light (Argyll Robertson pupils) and absence of knee jerks aid the diagnosis.

(iii) *Herpes zoster*. Pain and paraesthesia precede the rash by a few days. It is usually unilateral and segmental and should not really cause confusion.

(5) Psychiatric cause

Munchausen's syndrome. These patients present with convincing symptoms and signs of variable acute conditions often involving the abdomen, which may be covered with scars. When the patient is apprised of your suspicions, the symptoms and signs disappear and the patient rapidly takes his own discharge, usually resisting offers of psychiatric help.

MANAGEMENT

Implies excluding those conditions mentioned above. Obviously they will not all be relevant in every case of acute abdominal pain, but it is suggested that whenever possible the following investigations should be done:

(1) a plan x-ray of the abdomen, where possible erect and supine;
(2) chest x-ray;
(3) blood film;
(4) examine the urine for sugar, blood and pus cells;
(5) serum amylase;
(6) ECG.

PARALYTIC ILEUS

The following conditions should be borne in mind:

(1) drugs, e.g. ganglion blocking agents (especially mecamylamine and pentolinium) anti-Parkinsonian drugs and anticholinergic drugs (e.g. atropine);
(2) hypokalaemia;
(3) severe gastro-enteritis;
(4) certain spinal events, e.g. spinal fusion, prolapsed intervertebral disc and spinal fractures.

ACUTE GASTRIC DILATION

DIAGNOSIS

(1) May occur in hyperglycaemia, after childbirth, abdominal injury, application of a spinal cast and occasionally after abdominal surgery.
(2) The abdomen is distended and uncomfortable and a succussion splash can be readily elicited. Sufficient fluid may accumulate in the stomach to cause hypovolaemic shock.

(3) If reflux of the stomach contents occurs into the oesophagus the condition may be complicated by inhalation pneumonia.

MANAGEMENT

(1) Take blood for haemoglobin and PCV, electrolytes and urea.
(2) Pass a naso-gastric tube and empty the stomach. Usually more than 1·5 litres can be aspirated.
(3) Set up a drip, preferably with a central venous pressure line and replace the fluid lost into the bowel with alternating bottles of 5% dextrose and N saline. Add 26 mEq KCl to each litre of fluid given.
(4) Check the electrolytes six hours later and adjust the ratio of saline to dextrose and the potassium supplements in the usual way.
(5) If reflux of abdominal contents into the lungs occurs, large doses of steroids may minimise the ensuing inflammation. Give solumedrone 2 g i.v. daily for 2 days.

Acute liver failure[29,30]

DIAGNOSIS

(1) Should be considered in any confused (*see* p. 235) or unconscious (*see* p. 253) patient.

(2) May be caused by:

(i) Serious disease in a previously healthy patient; e.g. virus hepatitis, profound surgical shock with or without Gram-negative septicaemia, Weil's disease, paracetamol overdose, repeated halothane exposure or carbon tetrachloride poisoning. In this situation there are no signs of chronic liver disease, but there is an acute onset of progressive and severe encephalopathy associated with jaundice. You should look for clinical evidence of these viz;

(a) flapping tremor—demonstrated with the hands in dorsiflexion. More common, however, is generalised muscle twitching;
(b) hepatic foetor;
(c) constructional apraxia, restlessness, delusions or hallucinations;
(d) jaundice (which may appear only after your patient has become confused and delirious).

The mortality in this group is very high, particularly if coma has occurred.

(ii) A relatively minor stress to a patient with biochemical and clinical evidence of chronic liver disease. This is the commonest situation and may be precipitated by:

(a) gastro-intestinal haemorrhage (*see* p. 93);
(b) surgery;
(c) acute alcoholism;
(d) acute infection;
(e) potassium depletion and alkalosis (usually due to over vigorous use of diuretics);
(f) drugs—morphine, paraldehyde, short and medium acting barbiturates, acetazolamide and ammonium chloride (and *see* above);

110

    (g) paracentesis abdominis—ascitic fluid should be tapped in small quantities for diagnostic purposes; and only in large quantities for relief of symptoms;

    (h) constipation.

(3) Do not forget that the patient with cirrhosis may also get hyponatraemia due to the sick cell syndrome (*see* p. 113). There may also be features associated with the cause of the cirrhosis. This is particularly relevant in alcoholic cirrhosis. Here delirium tremens, thiamine deficiency producing Wernicke's encephalopathy, other B vitamin deficiencies and epileptic fits may all contribute to the disturbances in consciousness.

MANAGEMENT

Although the principles of management of acute and acute on chronic liver failure are similar, the objectives are somewhat different. In acute liver failure, support measures are used to buy time for the liver to regenerate and return to normal. In acute on chronic failure, however, the underlying damage will not usually be amenable to any specific therapy. Thus, measures appropriate to the management of acute liver failure may not always be appropriate in acute or chronic failure. Obviously decisions as to which measures are appropriate will be taken in the context of each individual case.

In all patients with liver failure take blood for full blood picture, electrolytes and urea, liver function tests including prothrombin time and plasma proteins, blood group, and blood glucose, blood cultures and plasma ammonia. Take arterial blood for blood gas measurements. Save serum for leptospira antibodies and Australia antigen, in case these become relevant later on. An EEG which shows progressive slowing of the alpha waves with increasing coma is a useful objective method for assessing developments.

Further management involves:

(1) General care of the confused (*see* p. 235) or unconscious (*see* p. 253) patient. Sedation should be avoided if at all possible (*see* (xii) below) but if you think sedation to be necessary give phenobarbitone 100 mg i.m., diazepam 5 mg i.v. or chlormethiazole (*see* p. 239). Drugs included in (2) (ii) (f) above must never be given.[27, 28]

(2) Treatment of the cause. Specific treatments are few, exceptions being chronic aggressive hepatitis (steroids) and Weil's disease (penicillin).

Steroids are sometimes given in fulminating virus hepatitis but they have not been shown to increase the survival rate.

(3) Stopping or treating the precipitating or contributory factors mentioned above.

(4) Minimising or correcting the multiple effects of liver cell failure:

    (i)   Minimising the protein load.[24] The rationale behind this is that the three groups of substances which appear in increased amounts in liver failure, and are the leading contenders for causing coma, are protein related metabolites.[25, 26] They are:

        (a) Ammonia. This arises largely through bacterial action on proteins in the gut, and is usually converted to urea by the liver. It causes coma in experimental animals, but not all patients dying of liver failure have a raised ammonia level.

        (b) Amines. Several amines, notably octopamine and phenylethanolamine, are present in increased amounts. It is conceivable that they act as false neurotransmitters in the brain.

        (c) Amino-acids. Amino-acid profiles are abnormal in liver disease. The amino-acid precursors of octopamine and phenylethanolamine are present in increased amounts which may account for the increased levels of these amines.

    Therefore give:

    (a) a low protein diet (20 g/day);

    (b) about 6·4 mJ (1500 kcal) as carbohydrate. This may be given either orally (e.g. 3–4 bottles of Hycal each of which contains 425 kcal) or intra-venously via a central venous catheter (e.g. 1200 ml of 33% dextrose);

    (c) sterilise the gut with neomycin 1 g four-hourly by mouth and lactulose in a dose just sufficient to cause diarrhoea and lower the faecal pH to below 6 (approx. 30 ml t.i.d.).

    (d) magnesium sulphate enemas as well as 60–180 ml of 50% magnesium sulphate by mouth as a purge.

    (ii)   Correcting fluid and electrolyte imbalance:

        (a) Do not give more than 2 litres of fluid per day.

(b) The serum sodium is usually low (120–130 mmol/1). If the patient is heavier than normal or if there is ascites or oedema this probably reflects dilution and redistribution rather than depletion. Giving sodium in this situation exacerbates fluid retention. The treatment is restriction of fluids to not more than 400 ml per day. Complaints of thirst from the patient can be alleviated by giving lemons to suck. However, with prolonged dietary sodium restriction and intensive diuretic therapy a true sodium depletion state can occur. (Serum sodium usually less than 120 mEq/l.) In this situation saline infusion may cause dramatic clinical improvement but should never be undertaken without getting expert advice. Dilutional hyponatraemia is by far the commoner of the two, and if there is doubt, saline should not be given. Terminally, sodium enters the cells causing a further drop in serum sodium. Do not attempt to correct this with hypertonic saline. The outlook at this stage is almost hopeless. 200 mg of hydrocortisone six-hourly and an infusion of glucose, potassium and insulin which helps to re-establish the sodium pump may be given (*see* p. 13).

(c) Potassium. Dangerous hypokalaemia can occur and potassium chloride supplements are given in the usual way.

(iii) Correction of coagulation defects.[23] These may arise for either of two reasons:

(a) Inadequate manufacture of clotting factors by the liver. This is only correctable by infusion of blood or blood products. Fresh frozen plasma (FFP) which contains all the clotting factors is the infusion of choice. If the platelet count is low, either a platelet infusion, or an infusion of fresh blood may be required. Vitamin K 15 mg i.m. should also be given, although theoretically it should not be of great value, unless there has been fat soluble vitamin malabsorbtion because of bile salt deficiency. If more than four units of ACD blood are necessary, give 10 ml 10% calcium gluconate/l of blood, as these patients are said to be particularly susceptible to citrate intoxication.

(b) Intravascular coagulation associated with acute hepatic necrosis. This can be recognised by the combination of bleeding tendencies and bruising, thrombocytopaenia, prolonged pro-thrombin, thrombin, and kaolin cephalin times, a low fibrinogen titre and raised titre of fibrinogen degradation products. IV heparin and fresh blood is the treatment of choice in this situation. This is clearly hazardous and should only be undertaken in conjunction with your haematological colleagues.

(c) Remember that every time you damage a blood vessel, bleeding is encouraged. Therefore, be sparing of your assaults on your patient.

(iv) Correcting the blood glucose:

(a) hypoglycaemia may occur. If this is present give 25 g of dextrose intravenously in the usual way and check the blood sugar by dextrostix four-hourly.

(b) Alternatively, hyperglycaemia may be present. This rarely needs treatment—unless ketosis develops. It is treated in the usual way with insulin (*see* p. 134).

(v) Correcting the effects of widespread peripheral dilation. This may cause hypotension and/or acute renal failure. Its mechanism is obscure, and treatment difficult. You should set up a central venous pressure line and ensure that the CVP is within the normal range (*see* p. 276). Then infuse dopamine, beginning at a dose of between 2 to 5 μg/kg/min and increasing as necessary to a dose of 20 μg/kg/min. At this level of infusion it causes vasoconstriction to all arteries except those in the brain and kidney.

(vi) Combating sepsis. Amoxycillin in the usual doses 250 mg i.v. eight-hourly is safe, but if gentamicin is used, blood levels should be monitored (*see* p. 248). Remember septicaemia is common in acute hepatic necrosis, whatever the cause.

(vii) Minimizing the occurrence of gastro-intestinal haemorrhage from acute erosions—give cimetidine 200 mg six-hourly i.v. in 5% dextrose, which will maintain the pH of the stomach contents above 6.

(viii) Supporting respiration. Many patients with acute hepatic failure develop shock lung (*see* p. 83). They may therefore require early ventilation to maintain an adequate PaO_2.

(ix) Cerebral oedema. There is experimental evidence in animals that massive doses of steroids delays the onset of cerebral oedema. As this complication is now the commonest cause of death in acute liver failure, we recommend giving dexamethasone 32 mg stat and 8 mg q.d.s. recognising that this is not of proven benefit in humans.[31]

(x) Lowering the concentration of circulating substances usually removed by the liver, e.g. ammonia. The following methods have been used.

(a) Exchange transfusion of about 10 units of heparinised blood. At the end of the exchange the heparin should be reversed by giving protamine. Alternatively, plasma exchanges may be undertaken. This involves taking blood and separating plasma from the red blood cells. The latter are returned together with fresh frozen plasma. This is equally time-consuming but does not tax the Blood Transfusion Service. Blood may be taken from the inferior vena cava and returned to a major vein. Alternatively, two lines of an arteriovenous Scribner shunt may be used, or access to a major artery and vein may be obtained by catheterisation, using the Seldinger technique;

(b) haemoperfusion over an activated charcoal column;

(c) haemodialysis;

(d) cross circulation;

(e) extra corporeal liver perfusion;

(b)–(e) can only be undertaken by specialist unit, whose advice should be sought. The purpose of using these various support measures is to buy time until adequate liver regeneration occurs. However, controlled trials have not shown any of these methods to be superior to conservative therapy

(xi) Liver transplantation continues in a few centres and may in time, be a feasible proposition for any of the 200–300 patients dying of acute liver disease in Britain each year.

(xii) Sedation. Patients with acute liver failure may become disorientated and violent for many reasons and you should ensure that there is no reversible cause, such as hypoxia, before using any sedation. If sedation is essential the benzodiazepam group of drugs are safest. Diazepam, 5 mg i.v. by slow intravenous infusion usually secures peace for all. As it is metabolised by the liver, the dosage should be kept as low as possible, and repeated as infrequently as possible.

SECTION III REFERENCES

Upper G.I. haemorrhage

1   Conn HO, Ramsby GR, Storer EH, *et al*. Intra-arterial vasopressin in the treatment of upper G.I. haemorrhage. *Gastroenterology* 1975; **68**: 211.

2   Finkelstein W. Cimetidine. *N Engl J Med* 1978; **299**: 992.

3   Forrest JAH. The investigation of acute upper gastro intestinal haemorrhage. *Br J Hosp Med* 1974; **12**: 160.

4   Foster DN, Miloszewski K, Losowsky MS. Diagnosis of Mallory-Weiss lesions. *Lancet* 1976; **2**: 483.

5   Hoare AM. Comparative study between endoscopy and radiology in acute upper gastro-intestinal haemorrhage. *Br Med J* 1975; **1**: 27.

6   Jick H, Porter J. Drug induced gastro-intestinal bleeding. *Lancet* 1978; **2**: 87.

7   La Brooy SJ, Misiewicz JJ, Edwards SJ, *et al*. Controlled trial of cimetidine in upper gastro-intestinal haemorrhage. *Gut* 1979; **20**: 892.

8   Leader. Identifying the cause of gastro-intestinal bleeding. *Lancet* 1971; **2**: 415.

9   Swain CP, Brown SG, Storey DW. Controlled trial of argon laser photocoagulation in bleeding peptic ulcers. *Lancet* 1981; **2**: 1313.

10 Conn HO. To scope or not to scope. *N Engl J Med* 1981; **304**: 967.

11 Leader. Erosive gastritis. *Br Med J* 1974; **3**: 211.

12 Leader. Prevention or cure for stress induced gastro-intestinal bleeding. *Br Med J* 1980; **2**: 631.

13 Macdougall BRD, Wetaby D, Theodossi A. Increased long term survival in variceal haemorrhage using injection sclerotherapy. *Lancet* 1982; **2**: 124.

14 Parbhoo S. The management of bleeding in liver disease. *Br J Hosp Med* 1975; **13**: 17.

15 Freeman JG, Cobden I, Lishman AH, Controlled trial of glypressin versus vasopressin in the early treatment of oesophageal varices. *Lancet* 1982; **2**: 66.

16 Pitcher LJ. Safety and effectiveness of the modified Sengstaken-Blakemore tube—a prospective study. *Gastroenterology* 1971; **61**: 291.

17 Allison DJ, Hemingway AP, Cunningham DA. Angiography in gastro-intestinal bleeding. *Lancet* 1982; **2**: 30.
18 Scott J, Dick R, Long RG, *et al*. Percutaneous transhepatic obliteration of gastro-oesophageal varices. *Lancet* 1976; **2**: 53.

Ulcerative colitis

19 Keighley MRB, Burrow DW, Arabi Y, *et al*. Randomised control trial of vancomycin for pseudomembranous colitis and post operative diarrhoea. *Br Med J* 1978; **2**: 1667.
20 Truelove SC, Jewell DP. Intensive intra-venous regime for severe attacks of ulcerative colitis. *Lancet* 1974; **1**: 1067.
21 Truelove SC, Willoughby CP, Lee EC, *et al*. Further experience in the treatment of severe attacks of ulcerative colitis. *Lancet* 1978; **2**: 1086.
22 Harvard C. Medical states simulating the acute abdomen. *Br J Hosp Med* 1972; **7**: 44.

Acute liver failure

23 Flute PT. Haemostasis in liver disease. *Br Med J* 1971; **1**: 215.
24 Hoyumpa AM, Desmond PV, Avant GR, *et al*. Hepatic encephalopathy. *Gastro-enterology* 1979; **76**: 184.
25 Leader. Biochemical monitoring of encephalopathy in liver disease. *Lancet* 1980; **2**: 783.
26 Leader. False neurotransmitters and hepatic failure. *Lancet* 1982; **1**: 86.
27 Leader. Safe prescribing in liver disease. *Br Med J* 1973; **2**: 193.
28 Leader. Sedation in liver disease. *Br Med J* 1977; **1**: 1241.
29 Leader. Heroic treatment for fulminant hepatic failure. *Br Med J* 1977; **2**: 1301.
30 Williams R. Treatment of fulminant hepatic failure. *Br Med J* 1971; **1**: 213.
31 Hanid MA, Davies M, Mellon PJ. Clinical monitoring of intracranial pressure in fulminant hepatic failure. *GUT* 1980; **21**: 866.

SECTION IV

ACUTE RENAL FAILURE

Acute renal failure [1,6,7,8] (ARF)

ARF may be defined as a sudden rise in urea with or without accompanying oliguria (less than 400 ml/24 hour in an adult). It is customary and helpful, to consider ARF as either:

(i)   Pre-renal.
(ii) Renal (established renal failure).
(iii) Post-renal.

(1) **Pre-renal**
A physiological response of the kidney to poor perfusion, which may be caused by:

(i)   hypovolaemia, the commonest situation. This may either be absolute, due to fluid or blood loss, or relative, as occurs for example in septicaemia, major overdoses, liver failure and pancreatitis;
(ii) cardiac failure.

In the initial stages of pre-renal failure, the kidneys' concentrating power is normal, and the urine produced is highly concentrated (*see* Table 1). It is essential to recognise this since restoring perfusion will avert established renal failure (ATN *see* below).

(2) **Renal**
Renal damage *per se* is characterised by considerable deterioration in renal function and concentrating power. The urine produced therefore, is dilute, and serves to distinguish renal from pre-renal failure (*see* Table I). Established renal failure may be due to:

(i)   Acute Tubular Necrosis (ATN). The mechanism underlying ATN is unclear, but it usually follows pre-renal failure.
(ii) Nephrotoxins.[4] These may be:

(a) Inorganic chemicals (e.g. mercuric chloride, phosphorus salts or heavy metals).
(b) Organic chemicals—carbon tetrachloride and ethylene glycol, for example.

121

TABLE I   Urine differences in pre-renal and established renal failure

	Pre-renal failure	Established renal failure
Urine/Plasma Osmolal ratio	>1·5:1	1·1:1
Urine/Plasma Urea ratio	>10:1	<4:1
Sodium mmol/1	<10	>20

    (c) Drugs—cephaloridine, colomycin, organic mercurials and phenindione have, amongst others, been implicated.

(iii) Acute glomerulonephritis. Either primary, or secondary to a systemic disease, such as SLE, PAN, or Henoch Schönlein purpura.

(iv) Haemolytic Uraemic Syndrome (HUS) including thrombotic, thrombocytopaenic purpura. Characterised by disseminated intravascular coagulation, which obliterates the renal capillaries, and micro-angiopathic haemolytic anaemia.

(v) Incompatible blood transfusions (*see* p. 246).

(vi) Hypercalcaemia (*see* p. 158).

(vii) Myeloma.

(viii) Acute or chronic failure. A trivial insult to a chronically diseased kidney may produce acute renal failure.

(3) Post-renal

Obstruction to urine flow, with consequent reduction in renal function, may occur in the:

(i) Tubules—Bence-Jones protein or myeloma para-protein, urate or sulphonamide crystals.

(ii) Ureter—calculi, retroperitoneal fibrosis, and tumours, most commonly of cervix or bladder. Bear in mind the possibility of obstruction to a single kidney.

(iii) Urethra—prostatic hypertrophy or urethral stricture.

    If the obstruction is relieved, prompt and rewarding return of renal function can be achieved.

DIAGNOSIS

The diagnosis of ARF, as defined, is biochemical. The signs and symptoms of uraemia, drowsiness, nausea and twitching are often overshadowed by the underlying cause.

(1) The history may give clues of longstanding renal disease, such as polyuria and nocturia and there may be stigmata of chronic renal failure such as hypertension, anaemia, pigmentation, pruritus, or renal bone disease with characteristic radiological changes of periosteal resorbtion of the distal phalanges. In such cases the kidneys, when visualised, may either be large (polycystic or hydronephrotic) or small and shrunken. If there has been no previous renal disease the kidneys are of normal size. In HUS there is an anaemia and thrombocytopaenia, and fragmented cells are seen in the blood film. Clotting factors are often normal.

(2) The biochemical changes usually present are:

   (i) *Raised urea*. ARF is usually accompanied by a catabolic state, and the urea deriving from excessive protein breakdown can only accumulate—serum creatinine is also raised to a relatively lesser degree.

   (ii) *Raised potassium*. Potassium, released from cells by acidosis, catabolism and the sick cell syndrome (*see* p. 113) accumulates and may cause fatal cardiac dysrhythmias.

   (iii) *Low sodium*. This is usually caused by fluid overload (dilution) or the sick cell syndrome (redistribution) as opposed to true sodium depletion.

   (iv) *Low HCO_3*. Metabolic acidosis is due to inadequate secretion of non-volatile anions (e.g. SO_4 and PO_4), inadequate renal tubular generation of HCO_3, and inadequate formation of NH_3 by the distal tubules. H^+ ion formation may also be increased in this situation by poor tissue perfusion, and tissue damage.

(3) Whatever the cause of ARF septicaemia is highly likely, as is circulatory overload and oedema from inappropriate fluid intake. Features of these conditions usually are clinically obvious.

MANAGEMENT

(A) Is aimed initially at diagnosing and correcting reversible or predisposing factors, i.e. poor renal perfusion or post-renal obstruc-

tion. If these measures do not restore renal function (i.e. established ARF is present) further aims are given below.

(B) Reducing the work load of the kidney by minimising tissue
breakdown and hypoperfusion.

(C) Dealing with the metabolic sequelae of kidney failure until renal
function is restored.

(D) Making a specific diagnosis of the cause of ARF and giving
appropriate therapy. This is not usually immediately relevant to
management, and will not be discussed further.

So

(1) Take blood for electrolytes, urea, FBP (including platelets) clotting factors, blood cultures, serum Ca^{++} and blood glucose. Send
urine, if necessary obtained by catheterisation, for Na^+ urea and
osmolarity (*see* Table I). This only requires a few millilitres of
urine, takes a short time to do, and must be insisted upon. Take a
straight x-ray of the abdomen to evaluate renal size and visualise
calculi.

(2) Weigh the patient if possible.

(3) Rule out a pre-renal cause.

(i)   Assess the patient for renal underperfusion. Heart failure
is usually obvious and requires conventional treatment.
Hypovolaemia causing general tissue under-perfusion
may also be evident clinically; i.e. cool peripheries,
tachycardia, hypotension (particularly postural hypotension), plus disturbances of consciousness. If there has been
substantial fluid loss, there may be reduced skin turgor and
eyeball tension will be low. A dry mouth and tongue is
significant only in the absence of mouth breathing. The
urine shows the characteristics of pre-renal failure. However, assessment of hypovolaemia can be extremely
difficult particularly if it is relative hypovolaemia, and if
there is any doubt the central venous pressure must be
measured (*see* p. 275). If this confirms hypovolaemia
appropriate fluid (saline, blood of plasma) must be given
rapidly until the CVP is in the upper range of normal (*see*
p. 277). Occasionally this manoeuvre restores urine flow
even when the urine has shown the characteristics of established renal failure, but in this situation restoration of
tissue perfusion must be carried out with the greatest
attention to signs of impending fluid overload.

(ii) If correction of hypovolaemia or obstruction does not lead to a brisk diuresis, renal damage has occurred, and established renal failure is present.

(iii) Remember that hypovolaemia may be due to a hypoproteinaemic state, such as the nephrotic syndrome, in which case circulating volume may be restored with either 1 litre of salt-free albumin or 1 litre of dextran 110.

(4) Rule out a post-renal cause:

(i) Catheterise the bladder to ensure that urethral obstruction is not present. If the bladder is empty, insert 200 ml of 0·02% solution of chlorhexidine, and withdraw the catheter.

(ii) Obstruction higher up may be difficult to exclude, but a high dose nephrotomogram, which is mandatory in ARF[3] (0·2 ml/kg body weight of 40% sodium diatrizoate) will usually demonstrate the presence of dilated pelvi-calyceal systems and must always be done to exclude obstruction. It will also show the size and number of kidneys. This is helpful because:

(a) small, possibly scarred kidneys indicate chronic renal disease;

(b) it is a necessary pre-requisite for renal biopsy which may be helpful diagnostically.

A high dose of IVU constitutes a large osmotic load, and may precipitate acute cardiac failure. Thus, metabolic and circulatory disturbances must be corrected before a high dose IVU is undertaken (*see* below). When obstruction is confirmed, the surgeons must be contacted without delay.

MANAGEMENT OF ESTABLISHED ARF

(1) *The precipitating condition* will need treatment on its own merits.

(2) (i) 50 ml of 25% mannitol, i.v. over 2 hours, or frusemide 500 mg i.v. over 1·5 hours may initiate a diuresis, and by promoting the polyuric phase of renal failure, curtail the duration of the illness.

(ii) Mannitol can precipitate acute cardiac failure in patients who are already overloaded; frusemide must never be given to patients who are still hypovolaemic, as it may reduce tissue perfusion still further.

(3) *Fluid balance*. Fluid intake should be 500 ml plus fluid lost the previous day (bearing in mind diarrhoea, vomiting and leaking fistulae). A weight loss of up to 0·5 kg/day indicates appropriate fluid replacement and is due to tissue loss. Gross fluid overload is an indication for dialysis.

(4) *Nutrition*. Starvation is the commonest cause for continuing catabolism in ARF and every attempt should be made to provide 12·6 mJ (3000 kcal) as carbohydrate or fat/day. This will reduce the urea load and promote healing. High calorie fluids such as Caloreen 16·7 kJ (4 kcal)/g or Hycal 1·0 mJ (244 kcal)/100 ml given with due attention to the necessity for fluid restriction, are suitable diets.

Twenty grams of protein/day is allowable in a low K^+, high carbohydrate, diet. Parentrovite forte 10 ml i.v. or equivalent should be given daily. Of course, if as is usually the case the patient is being dialysed a 60 g protein high calorie diet can be given, and constitutes one of the advantages of dialysis. IV fluids should only be given if oral feeding is impossible. A CVP line inserted with due regard to sterility helps, as the solutions you will infuse are highly irritant to small veins. Fifty per cent dextrose 4·2 mJ (1000 kcal)/500 ml, 10% Intralipid 2·1 mJ (550 kcal)/500 ml, are the most concentrated calorie sources and contain no electrolytes. IV feeding may induce acute carbohydrate intolerance (common anyway in ARF) and blood glucose levels should be checked regularly.

(5) *Potassium*. Is often high and may reach dangerous levels (more than 7 mmol) which require treatment.

(i)   Ten millilitres of 10% calcium chloride i.v. is the best emergency therapy. This decreases the excitability of membranes rather than actually reducing the serum K^+.

(ii) IV infusion of 500 ml 20% dextrose containing 25 units insulin over 2 hours will reduce serum K^+ temporarily.

(iii) If there is acidosis and the patient is not overloaded, 75–100 mmol $NaHCO_3$ i.v. over 2 hours will reduce serum K^+.

(iv) Ion-exchange resins, either orally or rectally, can be used for the less urgent situation. Calcium zeocarb 225 (15 g t.i.d.) is perhaps the best.

(6) *Sodium*. As discussed above, low serum Na usually indicates Na dilution and re-distribution and is not an indication for saline infusion. Unless there is gross loss of electrolytes none should be given in the oliguric phase of ARF. In practice, small quantities (less than 30 mmol of Na or K^+/day) are unavoidable if nourishing food is provided.

(7) *Acidosis*. It is rarely possible to correct the acidosis, aside from correcting tissue perfusion and oxygenation. Life threatening acidosis (or $pH<7·1$) is an indication for dialysis as $NaHCO_3$, the appropriate corrective fluid, will exacerbate fluid overload. $NaHCO_3$ may, of course, be given as part of any replacement fluid necessary (*see* p. 246).

(8) *Infections*. Many patients with ARF are septicaemic—common organisms, being *Ps. pyocyaneus*, *B. proteus*, *E. coli* and bacteroides. Before the results of the blood cultures are available it is wise to start a broad spectrum, preferably bactericidal antibiotic regime; e.g. ampicillin 500 mg six-hourly, and cloxacillin 250 mg six-hourly. If a change of antibiotics is indicated they may be used as follows:

   (i) Gentamicin or kanamycin are useful drugs but require monitoring of blood levels. Gentamicin given as loading dose of 5 mg/kg/24 hour in three instalments, is used initially. Further doses are given according to blood levels (*see* p. 248). Remember that frusemide enhances the toxicity of gentamicin. Kanamycin is given as a loading dose of 15 mg/kg/day given in three instalments. Peak blood levels (one hour after i.m. dosage) should be between 20–25 μg/ml.

   (ii) Cephalothin 6 g/day in divided doses or chloramphenicol 500 mg six-hourly may be used safely, and without blood level monitoring. Cefoxitin may also be used.

   (iii) Azlocillin, 4 g/day in two divided doses may be used.

   (iv) Fungal infections may supervene and should be looked for in blood cultures. The likely organism is *Candida*, acquired endogenously, and oral amphotericin lozenges 1 q.d.s. should be given prophylactically. For the treatment of candidal septicaemia (*see* p. 250).

   (v) If bacteroides is found metronidazole, chloramphenicol or clindamycin should be used (*see* pp. 249–50).

   (vi) Do not give tetracyclines as they raise the blood urea.

(9) *Drugs*. Many are excreted unchanged by the kidney. Before giving any drug to a patient in renal failure, make sure you know the appropriate dose. Drug levels are often available now—avail yourself of them. Maxolon 10 mg (1 ml) is a safe antiemetic, and diazepam a suitable sedative. Paracetamol is probably the safest mild analgesic to use. Pethidine and morphine can be used in normal dosage as necessary.

Scrutinise the drug sheet daily, as a deterioration in either renal function or the patient's general state may be drug related.

(10) *General*. The patient with ARF has a physically and psychologically debilitating illness. You must try and keep up his morale (yours as well). Keep him as mobile and active as possible. Always have a therapeutic reason for any invasive techniques both for his own peace of mind and for reasons of infection. Remember that the quality of nursing care is a major determinant of the ultimate outcome, and will be improved if the nurses understand what is happening (as much as you do).

(11) *Dialysis*. Haemodialysis or peritoneal dialysis facilitate control of uraemia, allow a more liberal diet, and tide the patient over whilst the kidneys recover.

Indications for dialysis are seldom absolute, but the following are general guidelines:

(i)   cardiac failure, or fluid overload, in an oliguric patient;
(ii)   serum K^+ greater than 7 mmol/1;
(iii) blood urea >50 mmol/1 (300 mg%);
(iv)   blood pH <7·1.

A deteriorating trend in your patient may require you to commence dialysis before the above figures are reached. The theory and practice of peritoneal dialysis, which can be carried out successfully in any general medical ward, is well described in 'Nephrology for Nurses'.[2]

SECTION IV REFERENCES

General

1   Black DAK. *Renal disease 3rd edition*. Oxford: Blackwell Scientific Publications, 1972.
2   Cameron SJ, Russell AME, Sale DNT, *et al. Nephrology for Nurses*. Heinemann Medical Examination Books, 1977.
3   Cattell WR, McIntosh CS, Moseley IF, *et al*. Excretion urography in acute renal failure. *Br Med J* 1973; **2**: 575.
4   Curtiss JR. Drug induced renal disorders. *Br Med J* 1977; **2**: 242.
5   Feest TG. Low molecular weight dextran—a continuing cause of ARF. *Br Med J* 1976; **2**: 1300.
6   Levinsky MJ. Pathophysiology of acute renal failure. *N Engl J Med* 1977; **296**: 1453.
7   Leader. Acute renal failure. *Lancet* 1973; **2**: 134.
8   Parsons V. Renal aspects of intensive care. *Br J Hosp Med* 1974; **11**: 843.

ENDOCRINE

Hyperglycaemic coma—ketotic[5]

DIAGNOSIS

(1) Usually presents itself with the gradual onset of polyuria and drowsiness (pre-coma) which may, over a day or more, progress to coma:

    (i) The patient usually shows signs of:

        (a) Sodium and water depletion—dry, slack skin tachycardia and hypotension, particularly posturally induced.

        (b) Acidosis—deep sighing respirations.

        (c) Ketosis—foetor and vomiting.

    (ii) The clinical picture is sometimes confused with salicylate poisoning which also shows reducing agents on Benedict's test. However, ketones, unlike salicylates, are volatile and are removed by boiling the urine.

    (iii) The predominant symptom of diabetic pre-coma may occasionally be abdominal pain, particularly in children. This and the finding of shifting areas of tenderness may obscure the signs of acidosis, ketosis and dehydration which are also usually present.

    (iv) The picture is utterly unlike that of hypoglycaemic coma. The only thing they have in common is that they may both occur in diabetes. If there is any doubt never give insulin. Instead give 50 g of glucose i.v. as a diagnostic test. This will do little harm to the patient in hyperglycaemic coma, whereas insulin can kill a hypoglycaemic patient or cause severe irreversible brain damage.

(2) Should be thought of in any patient drowsy or unconscious following:

    (i) surgery or other trauma;

    (ii) myocardial infarction;

    (iii) cerebral infarction.

(3) May be precipitated by an infection, which should always be looked for and treated as necessary.

(4) May rarely be caused by acute pancreatitis.

MANAGEMENT

If possible, the patient should be managed in an Intensive Care Unit.

(1) The aim of management is to correct:

    (i)   fluid loss—the average loss is 90–120 ml/kg;

    (ii)   electrolyte losses—especially potassium (average loss 3 mmol/kg) and sodium (average loss 7–10 mmol/kg);

    (iii) hyperglycaemia;

    (iv) acidosis.

(2) The fluid loss, causing hypovolaemia and the symptoms mentioned in (1) (i) above, should be corrected gradually (over the first 12 hours). Too rapid correction of hyperglycaemia causes gross osmotic swings, and too rapid correction of the acidosis causes large pH differences between the CSF and blood, both of which are potentially hazardous. So:

    (i)   Put up a drip. As in all hypovolaemic states a central venous pressure line is preferable, as it allows replacement of adequate (and often large) volumes of fluid with safety.

    (ii)   Take blood for electrolytes and urea, Hb and PCV and arterial pH. Check for ketonaemia by dipping a ketostix in plasma. This separates off the non-ketotic forms of diabetic acidosis (*see* below).

    (iii) Give i.v. fluids as quickly as possible until the CVP is normal and the patient is well perfused (usually 3–4 litres are necessary). Thereafter slow down the infusion rate to supply normal maintenance requirements and then keep the patient well perfused.

           Give the first 2 litres as 0·9% N saline and thereafter change to alternate bottles of 0·9% N saline and 5% dextrose. Potassium will also be required (*see* below).

    (iv) There are two commonly used regimes for giving insulin.[7] The easiest is to give a continuous low dose infusion of soluble insulin.[8] Make up 24 units of soluble insulin in 20 ml of N saline (*NOT* dextrose) and infuse at a dose of six units (5 ml of your solution)/hour. A constant infusion pump is ideal, but a paediatric giving set is a useful alternative. This dose of insulin causes an average fall in sugar of 4–5 mmol/hour. The rate of fall will be slower in the presence of infection. A less preferable regime is to give six units soluble insulin i.m. each hour, following a loading dose of 20 units i.m. It is unusual for patients to require more than six units of insulin per hour.

If they do, think of:

(a) infection;
(b) other endocrine problems, such as thyrotoxicosis or Cushing's syndrome;
(c) drug interaction; this is a particular problem in diabetic labour when very high doses—30 units i.v./hour—may be required to maintain normoglycaemia if dexamethasone or β-adrenergic agonists are being given.[9]

(3) Whilst this is going on:

Pass a urinary catheter. You will need this to ensure that an adequate urine flow is established (acute renal failure is very rare in diabetes possibly because the osmotic diuretic effect of glycosuria 'protects' the kidney). Do not rely on urine glucose to monitor progress—frequent blood glucose measurements are essential for this purpose. Remember to remove the catheter as soon as the patient is better (hopefully within 24 hours)—taking a catheter specimen of urine for culture as you do so.

(4) Next consider the following.

(i) *Electrolyte losses.* The polyuria preceding coma will have resulted in sodium and potassium depletion. Although the initial sodium is usually normal, the previous urinary losses have been hypotonic with respect to plasma. Hence, 5% dextrose may be given early in treatment (*see* (2) (iii) above). The initial plasma potassium may be high because of intracellular acidosis, but will fall rapidly as the blood glucose falls and as the acidosis is corrected. Thus, even if the initial potassium is high you are highly unlikely to run into problems with hyperkalaemia. The reverse is usually the case. One gram KC1 (13 mmol K^+) may be given with the first litre of fluid and the first dose of insulin provided the T waves on the ECG are not peaked, and, provided urinary output is adequate; 2 g KC1 (26 mmol K^+) given with each ensuing litre of fluid is usually sufficient. Occasionally even more may be required as shown by serial plasma K$^+$ estimations.

(ii) *Acidosis.* Although acidosis is itself dangerous the routine administration of HCO$_3$ to patients with a pH of more than 7·1 is not recommended because of the risk of:

(a) paradoxical increase in CSF acidosis alluded to above;
(b) further increasing K$^+$ flux into cells.
When the pH is less than 7·1 give 50 mmol of HCO$_3$ in the first 2 hours followed by 50 mmol in the next 4 hours.

Remember to give extra K$^+$.

(iii) *The precipitating cause.* Do an ECG, and if possible have a continuous ECG display to detect any arrhythmias or evidence of hyper or hypokalaemia. Look for infection, especially in the chest (chest x-ray) and urinary tract (urine microscopy and culture). Take blood cultures, routinely and start the patient on a broad spectrum antibiotic, such as ampicillin 500 mg q.d.s.

(iv) If your patient is comatose, aspirate the stomach contents through a naso-gastric tube, as many patients in diabetic coma have dilated, atonic stomachs, the contents of which may cause inhalation pneumonia. If there is no gag reflex, you should protect the lungs with a cuffed endotracheal tube prior to aspirating the stomach.

(v) Continuing hypotension is almost certainly due to hypovolaemia. If it persists despite adequate fluid replacement, consider other causes of hypotension (*see* p. 241) and treat accordingly.

(vi) General nursing care of the comatose patient (*see* p. 260).

(5) If you use the insulin regime suggested above, the blood glucose is likely to be halved within 4 hours—four-hourly estimates of blood glucose, electrolytes and arterial pH are therefore adequate.

(6) As a result of these and your other clinical measurements, you may have to adjust:

(i) *sodium*—by altering the ratio of 5% dextrose to N saline;
(ii) *potassium*—if the serum K$^+$ is normal, continue with the same dosage; if low, increase the dosage, and if high, stop

the K^+ immediately but take a further sample of estimation, as a high K^+ at this stage is extremely uncommon;

(iii) *bicarbonate*—if the pH is rising gradually, further administration of HCO_3 is unnecessary. If it is still dangerously low, i.e. less than 7·1, and not rising you may have to give more HCO_3. Give this slowly (i.e. 75 mmol in the next 4 hours).

(iv) *fluid*—you have probably not given the total replacement within 4 hours, but remember to watch the patient's neck veins and lung bases as well as the CVP to ensure you don't give too much.

(v) *PO_4*— hypophosphataemia of a significant degree (PO_4 <0·32 mmol/l) occasionally occurs in diabetic keto-acidosis. It causes general debility and energy, and may be corrected by infusing 9 mmol of monobasic potassium phosphate in 0·5% saline over 12 hours, and repeating as necessary.[5]

(7) Four hours later repeat the measurements. By now the patient should be considerably improved, and probably out of coma. If he is not:

(i) it may just be that the patient's initial metabolic disturbances were very severe, and are not yet corrected;

(ii) there may be an undetected precipitating cause of coma. Estimate the serum amylase and calcium at this stage, or before if there is a suggestive history of pancreatitis;

(iii) he may have one of the following complications of the condition or its treatment:

(a) *Hypoglycaemia*—check that the blood glucose is not below 4·5 mmol (80 mg%).

(b) *Cerebral oedema*[2] can occur;
—if too rapid lowering of blood glucose or,
—replacement of fluid loss with hypotonic solutions allows a high osmotic gradient to develop between extra and intra cellular compartments.

(c) *Hypokalaemia* and/or gastric dilation.

(d) *Major artery thrombosis*.

(e) *Addison's disease*—diabetic ketosis may precipitate an Addisonian crisis in a patient with pre-existing adrenal insufficiency. Check the arterial pressure.

(8) Improvement in blood sugar levels may precede improvement in other metabolic variables. Thus, the patient may be normo-glycaemic but still nauseated or vomiting. For this reason it is suggested that the insulin infusion rate should be reduced to three units per hour, and that 5% dextrose (1 litre over 8 hours) is given, as soon as the blood glucose is less than 11 mmol/l. This regime is continued until the patient can eat and drink normally. He should then start maintenance s.c. insulin. Assessing control by urine testing no longer has a place in the management of acute diabetic emergencies, and regimes of the sort outlined above are probably the easiest way of controlling any diabetic who cannot eat and drink e.g. those undergoing surgery or labour.

(9) Remember that the gross desalination of hyperglycaemia can mask signs of infection. These may become apparent when your patient's fluid deficiencies have been corrected, so always re-examine the patient carefully at this stage.

Hyper-osmolar non-ketotic diabetic coma[1,3,4,6]

(1) Diabetic coma may occur without ketonuria in the following circumstances:

    (i)   When diabetic coma is complicated by acute renal failure. Here the patient has ketonaemia and is acidotic.

    (ii)   Diabetic coma with lactic acidosis (*see* p. 143).

    (iii) Hyper-osmolar non-ketotic diabetic coma. These patients have no ketones in the urine or blood, are not acidotic and do not, therefore, overbreathe.

(2) In (1) (iii) above the patients frequently are elderly and have an insidious onset of illness over weeks. They may present with either focal or diffuse neurological signs with or without an accompanying cerebrovascular accident. The blood glucose is often very high (around 60 mmol) causing an osmotic diuresis in which large amounts of potassium, sodium and water are lost. The ensuing hypovolaemia is usually obvious clinically and is associated with pre-renal uraemia. There is proportionately greater loss of water than salt, and the serum sodium is often raised—above 155 mmol. The combination of a raised sodium, urea and glucose causes very high serum osmolality, which may exceed 400 mosmol/kg. This in turn causes severe intracellular dehydration—one of the factors responsible for coma.

(3) The pathogenesis of this illness is not fully established, but recent evidence suggests that these patients may have just sufficient circulating insulin to prevent lipolysis and thus prevent the development of ketones but not enough to prevent hyperglycaemia.[6] The prior use of thiazide diuretics which have an additional hyperglycaemic effect, is common.

MANAGEMENT

Take blood for haemoglobin and PCV electrolytes and urea, blood, glucose, serum amylase and calcium and plasma osmolality.

(1) Correct:

  (i)   Dehydration, hyperosmolality and sodium and potassium
         depletion. As mentioned in (2) above, the fluid and elec-
         trolyte loss in hyperosmolar coma is usually greater than
         that in ketotic coma. An average loss of 25% of the total
         body water is common. You should aim to replace half this
         loss in the first 12 hours, and the rest in the ensuing 24
         hours. The problem is with what. As so often, there is
         controversy. Some experts advocate using the same fluid
         and electrolyte regime as in ketotic diabetic coma (*see*
         p. 134). However, the conventional advice is to replace
         the water and sodium deficit with 0·5 N saline from the
         onset. Potassium supplementation is as for diabetic ketotic
         coma. A sensible compromise is to use 0·5 N saline if the
         initial serum sodium is above 155 mmol/l, or if the sodium
         rises above 155 mmol/l at any stage during treatment, but
         otherwise to give 0·9 normal saline as for ketotic coma.
         Remember when calculating fluid deficits that in old
         people, the total body water is only 50%, not the more
         usual 60%, of body weight.

  (ii)   Hyperglycaemia. It might be thought that the lack of
         acidosis allows full sensitivity to insulin. This is often, but
         by no means always, the case. Insulin should be given as
         described for ketotic diabetic coma, the response being
         checked with repeated measurements of the blood
         glucose.

(2) Venous and arterial thromboses are very likely to occur in this
    situation, so heparinise the patient for 2–3 days (10 000 units i.v.
    six-hourly).

(3) Treatment of any underlying or precipitating causes, such as
    infection or acute pancreatitis.

(4) After the acute episode has passed these patients often have mild
    diabetes which can be controlled with diet alone or small doses of
    oral hypoglycaemic agents.

Non-ketotic diabetic acidosis

The acidosis of diabetic pre-coma and coma is not always caused by ketones. It may occasionally be due to other anions; formic acid in methyl alcohol poisoning; alpha keto-glutaric acid in liver failure; phosphate and other anions in renal failure; and lactic acid. For this reason it is important to check that ketones are actually present in the plasma of a patient suspected of having diabetic ketosis. If they are absent then these other serious underlying conditions should be looked for.

Acute lactic acidosis[10]

Lactic acid is in equilibrium with pyruvate, the position of equilibrium being determined mainly by the tissue pO_2.

The lactate level, normally less than 1 mmol/l, will rise in the following circumstances:

(1) With a rise in the pyruvate concentration. Here the pyruvate lactate ratio is normal (1:10) and the patient is not acidotic. For reasons that are not understood this occurs in the setting of hyperventilation such as may occur after a stroke or pulmonary embolus for instance. The prognosis for these patients is that of their underlying disease, which should be treated in the normal fashion.

(2) With poor tissue oxygenation. Here lactate has risen ten times or more relative to pyruvate, and the patient is acidotic. There are two separate categories:

   (i) The decreased tissue oxygenation may be evident. The patient is seriously ill. The oxygen supply to the tissue is severely compromised, as in septic, cardiac or hypovolaemic shock, or hypoxia for any reason. In this group the excess blood lactate falls with therapy directed at reversing the underlying 'shock' state. (This group is the type A lactic acidosis of Cohen and Wood.)

   (ii) Lactate production may be increased, or lactate removal decreased without any obvious oxygen supply problems. Thus, the patient initially appears to be well perfused, with a normal Pao$_2$ and the reason for this lactate disturbance, despite an apparently adequate oxygen supply, is not clear. In this group of patients (type B lactic acidosis of Cohen and Wood), there may be no obvious antecedent illness, but more commonly there is an identifiable provocative factor. The most important of these are that the patient may have been taking phenformin, suffer from ethanol intoxication, have had a rapid sorbitol or fructose infusion, or have severe liver disease. Occasionally the acidosis develops in patients who seem to be recovering satisfactorily from an event such as a myocardial infarct.

142

In this group, the serum lactate levels are uninfluenced by oxygen therapy, and the serum bicarbonate often fluctuates wildly, and with apparently only little relation to HCO_3 infusion.

DIAGNOSIS

(1) Lactic acidosis should be suspected in acidotic (and therefore hyperventilating) patients if a large number of anions remain unaccounted for (the anion gap). The sum of the anions (Cl^- and HCO_3^-) normally approximates to the sum of the serum cations ($Na^+ + K^+$). Thus, if the anion gap $(Na^+ + K^+) - (Cl^- + HCO_3^-)$ is greater than 18 mmol/1, and is not accounted for by ketones, salicylates or ureamia, lactic acidosis may well be present.

(2) The presence of lactic acidosis should, of course, be suspected in a diabetic patient who is acidotic but who has no, or only few, circulating ketones.

(3) It has been noted that the PO_4 level is usually high in lactic acidosis. An average level of 2·9 mmol/l has been recorded, whereas in the metabolic acidosis of diabetic coma, the average is 1·6 mmol/l.

MANAGEMENT

Type A lactic acidosis

The excess lactate here is only one of degree, as most 'shock states' are accompanied by increased lactate levels. The treatment is that of the 'shock state' underlying the problem (*see* p. 242).

Type B lactic acidosis

This involves:

(1) Investigation for any underlying conditions. Include a full blood count, electrolytes and urea, blood culture, blood glucose, serum amylase and calcium, ECG, microscopy and culture of urine and arterial blood gases. Blood should be taken for grouping, and serum saved for cross matching. Unsuspected hypovolaemia

may be revealed by a low central venous pressure. A drug history will reveal that phenformin has been consumed.

(2) Treatment of the underlying condition is obviously of prime importance.

(3) Correction of the acidosis. Acidosis has a negative inotropic effect, and persistent acidosis will lead to shock and eventual death. It thus seems rational to treat the acidosis vigorously and early, in an attempt to halt this progression. Several measures have been advocated, although none has been subjected to a controlled trial.

  (i) Infuse isotonic (1·26%) $NaHCO_3$ at a rate sufficient to bring the blood pH up to normal within 2–6 hours, and then to keep it there. You will probably need between 600 and 1500 mmol $NaHCO_3$ to achieve this.

  (ii) Methylene blue 5 mg/kg given as an infusion to buffer excess lactate.

  (iii) Haemodialysis and peritoneal dialysis have both been used, without any great enthusiasm or success.

  (iv) Dichloroacetate. This is a powerful activator of pyruvate dehydrogenase, and induces a striking decrease in lactate concentration. It is not available for intravenous use, and is still under investigation, but use of the oral capsule (3·0 gm in a single dose each day) is promising.

(4) Hypoxaemia should be corrected using 50–60% O_2 by face mask.

Hypoglycaemic pre-coma and coma[13]

DIAGNOSIS

(1) Hypoglycaemia must be considered in any disorientated, aggressive or excitable person.

(2) Hypoglycaemia may be precipitated by alcohol, among other things. This mixture may be a difficult diagnostic problem to grapple with (sometimes literally) and is of medico-legal significance.

(3) Coma is an emergency *par excellence*. Minutes count if irreversible brain damage is to be prevented. It is characterised by a moist skin, dilated pupils, and possibly tachycardia.

(4) The significance of these signs may not strike the observer and hypoglycaemia must be considered and excluded in any unconscious patient. BM stix are adequate for this purpose and if they show a glucose content of less than 2·3 mmol/l (40 mg/100 ml) treatment should be given without waiting for the blood glucose result, for which blood should be taken first.

(5) The only thing that hypoglycaemic coma and hyperglycaemic coma have in common is that in both, the patient may be diabetic and unconscious. BM stix reliably distinguish the two. If you are still doubtful give dextrose i.v. (*see* below). It will do little harm to a patient in hyperglycaemic coma and will restore consciousness in patients with hypoglycaemic coma.

(6) Occasionally hypoglycaemia may present with focal neurological signs such as hemiplegia (p. 172).

(7) NEVER give insulin as a diagnostic test. In hypoglycaemia it is usually fatal and invariably disastrous.

MANAGEMENT

(1) Take blood for blood glucose, before initiating any treatment.

(2) If the patient can drink give 25 g dextrose in orange juice.

(3) If the patient is comatose, give 25 g dextrose i.v. (50 ml of 50% dextrose) and when the patient rouses, a further 25 g to drink.

(4) Glucagon may be given:

   (i)   If the patient cannot be restrained for long enough to give an i.v. injection safely, give glucagon 1 mg i.m., which raises blood sugar to within the normal range in 5–10 minutes.

(ii)   Sulphonylureas reduce hepatic release of glucose, probably as a consequence of their effect on raising insulin levels. The insulin antagonist action of glucagon may help reverse this process, and so glucagon should be used in any patient whose hypoglycaemia is induced by sulphonylureas.

(5)   Recovery is usually complete in 10 to 15 minutes but may take up to one hour occasionally, despite adequate blood glucose levels.

(6)   When the crisis is over consider the cause.[13]

(7)   In patients rendered hypoglycaemic by long-acting insulins, or whom you suspect of taking really large doses of any insulin, after you have undertaken the initial therapy as outlined above, you should put up a 10% dextrose drip, and keep this running for at least 24 hours, more often longer. This is to arrest the real danger of hypoglycaemia recurring over the ensuing 24–48 hours. The same strictures, apply to hypoglycaemia induced by the sulphonylureas. The blood sugar, as monitored by B.M. Sticks, should be maintained between 5 and 7 mmol/l.

Hypopituitary coma[14]

DIAGNOSIS

(1) May be precipitated in a patient with long-standing pituitary failure by infection, trauma (including surgery) myocardial infarction or cold, sedatives and hypnotics. It may also occur following an acute insult to the pituitary gland, e.g. surgery, head injury, haemorrhage or post-partum infection.

(2) The clinical picture is one of gonadotrophin, thyroid and adrenal deficiency.

These deficiencies have usually developed gradually, as have the patient's symptoms. Thus, there is a history of somnolence, sensitivity to cold and increasing confusion, progressing over a few weeks to coma. On examination, the skin is strikingly pale and dry, but of fine texture. Pubic and axillary hair is usually absent and the prematurely wrinkled features of hypogonadism may be obvious. The breasts and genitalia are atrophic. There is a general lack of pigmentation, and blood pressure temperature and pulse rate are often below normal. If in addition, the posterior pituitary is involved, polyuria due to a lack of ADH may cause dehydration.

These multiple endocrine deficiencies all contribute to the coma, as indicated below.

MANAGEMENT

Estimate the blood glucose with BM stix and take blood for full blood count, electrolytes and urea, blood glucose, serum thyroxine, blood cortisol and blood gases.

(1) Consider treatment of the possible causes of coma, of which the most common are:

    (i) *Hypothyroidism*. Attempts to raise the metabolic rate with tri-iodothyronine (T_3) whilst other causes of coma are still operative exacerbates coma, and this should not be given until treatment of other causes of coma is under way. A suitable regime for the administration of T_3 is:

147

0·02 mg eight-hourly for three doses;
0·05 mg eight-hourly for three doses;
0·1 mg eight-hourly thereafter.

The drug is most usually given via a naso-gastric tube, but can be given intravenously if the appropriate preparation is available.

(ii) *Hypothermia* (*see* p. 229).

(iii) *Electrolyte disturbances*. Two patterns of electrolyte disturbance may occur.

(a) *Water intoxication*. This is by far the most common, and arises because, in the absence of cortisol, the patient's capacity to mount a water diuresis is depressed. If the posterior pituitary is intact, the inappropriate secretion of ADH associated with myxoedema may also be a factor. Water intoxicated patients may complain of weakness, headache, nausea and blurring of vision. Tendon reflexes are exaggerated and muscle cramps occur. Drowsiness progresses to confusion, convulsions and coma. The serum sodium is usually less than 120 mmol/l, there may be hypokalaemia, and the urea is usually low (below 6·0 mmol/l). Intake of all fluids should be stopped, unless there is oliguria. This is frequently all that is necessary. However, if oliguria is present, if the patient is in pre-coma, or convulsions have occurred, give 2 N saline at about 40 ml/hour until the urine flow has been more than 45 ml/hour for at least 3 hours.

Because of the risk of water intoxication, you should not give hypotonic fluids to patients in hypopituitary coma until adequate replacement of cortisol and thyroxine has been achieved.

(b) *Salt and water depletion*. This is uncommon. The serum Na^+ may be low, but the urea will be high and the patient hypovolaemic. When it is due to polyuria secondary to ADH deficiency, give 5 units of aqueous pitressin subcutaneously and sufficient N saline to make good previous salt losses. However, it is more commonly due to vomiting and diarrhoea occurring in a patient with cortisol deficiency. N saline infusions will again be required.

(iv) A central venous pressure line will help considerably in the management of these electrolyte disturbances and you should insert one whenever possible.

(v) *Hypoglycaemia*. Give 25 g of dextrose i.v. (*see* p. 145).

The problems in (iii) and (v) are primarily caused by adrenocortical insufficiency and at least 100 mg of hydrocortisone must be injected i.v. without delay (*see* p. 152). This may initiate a diuresis if water intoxication has occurred, or protect the patient from water intoxication if saline and water depletion require large volumes of intravenous fluid. In addition the following may be contributory.

(vi) *Hypoxia*. Give 50–60% oxygen by face mask. If this is inadequate as judged by the Pao_2 intermittent positive pressure respiration is indicated.

(vii) *Hypotension*. This is usually due to steroid insufficiency and/or hypovolaemia and responds to hydrocortisone and adequate fluid replacement.

(2) Investigation and treatment of the cause.

(3) When coma has been relieved and the crisis is passed, daily replacement therapy will be necessary (*see* references).

(4) Diabetics who have been hypophysectomised for treatment of diabetic retinopathy are extremely sensitive to insulin—changes of a few units either way may lead to severe hypoglycaemia or ketoacidosis.

PITUITARY APOPLEXY

Pituitary apoplexy occurs when sudden haemorrhage and/or necrosis cause sudden expansion of a pituitary tumour.

DIAGNOSIS

(1) Presents with a characteristic array of symptoms and signs. There is a sudden onset of headache, bilateral amblyopia and ophthalmoplegia. The patient becomes stuporous and may lapse into coma. Neck stiffness may be present.

(2) A lumbar puncture should not be performed as this presentation is also consistent with a temporal lobe pressure cone.

(3) Skull x-ray nearly always shows enlargement of the sella.
(4) CT scan of the head may show parasellar haemorrhage and suprasellar mass effect.

MANAGEMENT

Since the patient may die within hours, neurosurgical help should be sought urgently. The relief of pressure by a transnasal decompression of the sella is the procedure of choice. In the interval give dexamethasone 6 mg i.v. every 6 hours together with the usual measures as necessary to support circulation and ventilation.

Addisonian crisis

INTRODUCTION

Addisonian crisis may be primary, due to destruction or atrophy of the adrenal gland, or secondary due to failure of the hypothalamic–pituitary–adrenal axis. The usual cause of secondary hypoadrenalism is the previous administration of exogenous steroids. Since theoretically only the glucocorticoid secretion is under pituitary control, mineralocorticoid deficiency should occur in primary but not in secondary hypoadrenalism. In fact, there is a tendency for the whole adrenal cortex to atrophy after long-term steroid ingestion, and mineralocorticoid deficiency may be assumed to be present in secondary hypoadrenalism.

DIAGNOSIS

(1) Should be considered in any hypotensive patient, who may also be vomiting, especially if they have received steroids within the past year. The signs of chronic adrenal insufficiency may or may not be present, so do not necessarily expect a pigmented, asthenic patient.
(2) It may be precipitated by infection, myocardial or cerebral infarction, trauma (including surgery), parturition or any metabolic stress. It may complicate septicaemia caused by pyogenic organisms—usually the meningococcus and is said to be due to haemorrhage into the adrenals. However, the majority of these patients are probably suffering from bacterial shock, for the plasma cortisols when measured are usually appropriately high.
(3) It is a useful, if cynical, maxim that in the above situation no one should be allowed to die with unexplained hypotension or coma without first receiving 200 mg of hydrocortisone i.v.

MANAGEMENT

The patient is depleted of sodium, potassium and water and may be hypoglycaemic. Take blood for baseline haemoglobin and PCV electrolytes and urea, blood glucose and plasma cortisol, then:

(1) Steroid replacement.

Give 100 mg hydrocortisone sodium succinate i.v. and 100 mg i.m. and then 50 mg i.m. eight-hourly. Although hydrocortisone is essentially a glucocorticoid it has sufficient mineralocorticoid activity when used in the above dosage to make it the drug of choice in both primary and secondary adrenal failure. However, some authorities suggest that a mineralocorticoid, such as deoxy-corticosterone 10 mg i.m. should be given in any case where there is profound hypotension or clinical shock.

(2) Estimate blood glucose by BM stix. If less than 2·3 mmol/l (40 mg%) give 25 g of glucose orally or i.v. without waiting for the blood sugar results.

(3) Put up a drip, preferably with a CVP line. Give at least 1 litre of N saline in 2 hours and then as necessary to keep the CVP within the normal range.

(4) Consider the cause:

   (i)   Do an ECG which may demonstrate myocardial infarction or hypokalaemia.

   (ii) Look for signs of infection. Do not start a broad spectrum antibiotic as a routine. However, if the patient is pyrexial without obvious cause investigations should include a chest x-ray, urine microscopy and blood cultures and then start on a broad spectrum antibiotic parenterally. Bear in mind that hyperpyrexia does occur occasionally as a feature of Addisonian crisis.

(5) By now the electrolyte results should be available:

   (i)   hyponatraemia needs further treatment with normal saline;

   (ii) potassium supplements may be necessary;

   (iii) further fluid replacement will depend on how much salt and water depletion has occurred. The commonest cause of continuing hypotension is hypovolaemia. Therefore, if in doubt set up a central venous pressure line and replace accordingly (*see* p. 277).

(6) Repeat the blood electrolytes and blood glucose after 4 hours and continue repeating the electrolytes eight-hourly if rapid fluid replacement is necessary. Water intoxication can easily occur in these patients if hypotonic saline is given and the serum sodium should not be allowed to fall below 125 mmol/l.

Myxoedema coma15,19,20,21

DIAGNOSIS

(1) Patients usually present during the winter months being particularly susceptible to hypothermia. It may, therefore, complicate conditions where hypothermia is common—such as strokes or chlorpromazine overdose.

(2) Before coma supervenes the patient may have been mentally dulled or psychotic.

(3) Usually the patient has the classical appearance and signs of myxoedema, except the delayed relaxation time of deep tendon reflexes which cannot be elicited. Hypotension and bradycardia are invariable.

(4) If coma has occurred, two-thirds of patients die. This may be due to insufficient appreciation of the multiple causes ((i) to (vii)) of coma.

(5) Onset of coma may be accompanied by convulsions which are treated in the usual way (see p. 182).

MANAGEMENT

(1) Measure blood glucose with BM stix and take blood for full blood count, electrolytes and urea, blood glucose, cortisol, T_4 or T_3 resin uptake and blood gases.

(2) Treat:

(i) *Hypothyroidism*. Whether to give tri-iodothyronine (T_3) or thyroxine (T_4) or both, and how much of each you should give is a subject steeped in controversy. The effect of T_3 begins in 4 hours or so, whereas T_4 takes longer to act. However, T_4 replacement is easier and more reliable, and its action is smoother. We think a reasonable policy is to give both, as outlined below.

(a) Tri-iodothyronine (T_3). Give 20 μg eight-hourly either by naso-gastric tube, or i.v. if a suitable preparation is available;

(b) In addition, give thyroxine (T_4) 200 μg i.v. stat and then 100 μg i.v. daily thereafter. The dosage of both the above should be halved if you are confident that your patient is suffering from ischaemic heart disease.

(ii) *Hypoadrenalism.* This will be present in all cases of myx-oedemic coma associated with hypopituitarism. As the pituitary status in any given patient with myxoedema coma may not be known, all should be given 100 mg hydrocor-tisone i.v. stat and then 50 mg i.m. eight-hourly.

(iii) *Hypoventilation.* This may give rise to hypoxia alone or hypoxia and hypercarbia. Measure the blood gases. If the $Paco_2$ is raised ($>$40 mmHg) ventilation will be required; ventilation may also be required if the Pao_2 cannot be kept above 60 mmHg with oxygen via a face mask.

(iv) *Hypothermia.* Do not warm the patient rapidly. This may cause cardio-vascular collapse. Simply use lots of blankets (*see* p. 229).

(v)   *Hypoglycaemia.* If this is present give 25 g of dextrose i.v. as frequently as necessary.

(vi) *Hypotension.* If the above measures do not restore the blood pressure give plasma expanders—blood, dextran 70 or plasma, whichever is available. If hypotension persists after hypovolaemia is corrected, as verified by a central venous pressure line, it may be necessary to use an isop-renaline infusion (*see* p. 245).

(vii) *Hyponatraemia.* This is nearly always caused by dilution and re-distribution, possibly due to inappropriate ADH secretion. The appropriate treatment is fluid restriction. Attempts to correct hyponatraemia by hypertonic saline infusions merely exacerbates fluid retention. However, if the serum sodium is less than 120 mmol and the patient is not oedematous, it is possible that hyponatraemia may be contributory to the coma. In this situation give 50 ml increments of 5 N saline hourly (65 ml) and watch the central venous pressure, lung bases and the effect on the serum sodium carefully.

Thyrotoxic crisis[18,19]

DIAGNOSIS

(1) The signs of breathlessness, anxiety, tremor, severe eye lid retraction and uncontrolled atrial fibrillation are virtually diagnostic. The thyroid gland is usually enlarged and obviously hyperactive.

(2) However, patients can occasionally present with:

    (i)   a rapidly progressive weakness leading to drowsiness and coma;

    (ii)   an acute psychosis;

    (iii) abdominal pain and vomiting, simulating an acute abdominal crisis.

(3) It is usually precipitated by an infection, surgery, diabetic ketosis, or by prematurely stopping anti-thyroid treatment. It may occasionally occur following ^{131}I therapy for thyrotoxicosis, if the gland has not been suppressed beforehand with iodine.

MANAGEMENT

Take blood for a full blood picture, electrolytes, blood glucose, and serum thyroxine, and save serum for tri-iodothyronine estimation should this be required later.

(1) *Hyperthyroidism*. Give:

    (i)   potassium iodide 600 mg i.v. over 1 hour and then 2 g orally per day. This is reduced when the hyperthyroidism comes under control and its beneficial effect lasts not longer than two weeks;

    (ii)   propylthiouracil, 1000 mg/day, or carbimazole 100 mg/day by mouth (or stomach tube if necessary) in three divided doses.

(2) *Anxiety*. If possible the patient should be nursed by himself in a quiet semi-dark room. Give:

(i) chlorpromazine 100 mg i.v. This also helps treat hyper-pyrexia;

(ii) if anxiety is severe an acute psychosis may supervene, which although sometimes resistant to chlorpromazine, usually responds to propranolol. The usual dose is 40 mg orally t.d.s. but it may be given i.v. 0·5–2 mg six-hourly if the patient is too sick to swallow. This may, however, precipitate severe hypotension and heart failure and propranolol should not be used if there is pulmonary or peripheral oedema unless there is associated atrial fibrilla-tion (*see* (3) below).[17] In the absence of heart failure it is wise to start with the lower dose increasing as necessary. Should heart failure supervene atropine 0·4–1·0 mg i.v. should be given.

(3) *Left ventricular failure.* This is caused by uncontrolled atrial fibrillation which is treated along the usual lines with diuretics and oxygen (*see* p. 34). In addition propranolol, in the dosage described above rapidly reduces the ventricular rate and restores sinus rhythm, thereby controlling the failure. Digoxin has no influence on the ventricular rate in this situation but is given as it increases the force of myocardial contraction. In atrial flutter propranolol is theoretically dangerous.

(4) *Hyperpyrexia.* Some degree of fever is always present and does not necessarily indicate infection. Use fans, and tepid sponge, together with chlorpromazine as above. Aspirin increases the metabolic rate, displaces thyroxine from pre-albumin, and should not be used. If the above measures are ineffective prop-ranolol given as above may cause dramatic improvement.

(5) *Dehydration.* This may occur from hyperventilation and sweat-ing as well as insufficient fluid intake. CVP recordings are especially valuable in this situation as hypovolaemia may be complicated by heart failure. Give 20% or 33% dextrose i.v. as extra calories are needed to supply increased metabolic demands. In addition, cautious replacement of sodium losses will also be necessary. Do not attempt to raise the serum sodium by giving hypertonic saline as this may precipi-tate pulmonary oedema. Repeat the electrolytes after 12 hours.

(6) *Adrenal insufficiency.* Hypotension and vomiting may be due to adrenocortical insufficiency which is unmasked by the metabolic stress. Take blood for plasma cortisol and give

100 mg of hydrocortisone i.v. without waiting for the result, followed by 50 mg six-hourly.

(7) *Thrombo-embolic complications.* These appear to be common, and serious. Give heparin (*see* p. 14).

(8) *Thyrotoxic crisis.* This may be fatal and in severe cases it may be necessary to anaesthetise, paralyse and ventilate the patient in an attempt to reduce metabolic requirements.

(9) The use of haemoperfusion over a polyacrylamide gel column has been advocated in intractable thyrotoxic crisis. This technique looks promising and is worth considering.[16]

(10) Effective therapy of the precipitation cause is a major determinant of the ultimate outcome.

Acute hypercalcaemia[23,25]

This may be caused by hyperparathyroidism, vitamin D intoxication, widespread bone metastases, non-metastatic complications of malignancies, the milk-alkali syndrome, myeloma or sarcoidosis (for differentiation see references[22]).

DIAGNOSIS

Disorders of behaviour, polydypsia, polyuria, vomiting and pyrexia may progress to cardiovascular collapse and coma. Acute renal failure, due in part to hypovolaemia, may occur. A fatal cardiac arrhythmia may terminate the condition. The serum calcium in these cases is usually more than 4 mmol (16 mg/100 ml).

Conjunctivitis due to corneal calcification seen as a gritty deposit on the corneo-scleral junction is the most striking physical sign. It is best seen with a hand lens and strong lateral lighting. The ECG shows a short QT interval.

MANAGEMENT

(1) Take blood for haemoglobin, PCV, electrolytes (including Cl^-) and urea, serum calcium, phosphate and alkaline phosphatase and plasma proteins.

(2) Replace fluid loss with isotonic saline and 5% dextrose giving potassium supplements as necessary—a CVP line is valuable.

(3) Lower the serum calcium. There are several ways of doing this:

    (i) Frusemide 100 mg/hour. This reduces the serum Ca^{++} by a mean value of 0·75 mmol (3·1 mg/ml) over 24 hours. The considerable fluid, Na^+, K^+ and Mg^{++} losses should be measured frequently and replaced. This requires intensive care, but provided adequate attention is paid to correcting the fluid and electrolyte loss, it is a safe and effective way of lowering Ca^{++}.

    (ii) Mithramycin 25 μg/kg i.v. over 3 hours in a solution of 5% dextrose or by a bolus. This is usually effective within 12–36 hours.

(iii) A traditional but inconvenient method has been to use a solution of sodium phosphate buffer pH 7·4 (81 mmol Na_2HPO_4 and 19 mmol NaH_2PO_4 made up to 1 litre with 19 mmKCl added). The solution should be infused over 8 hours, and has its maximum effect between 14 and 20 hours. The amount you give can be assessed from the following data:

  100 mm sodium phosphate (i.e. 1 litre of solution) infused over 8 hours gives a mean Ca^{++} depression of 1·5 mmol (6·1 mg/100 ml).

  75 mm sodium phosphate infused over 8 hours gives a mean serum Ca^{++} depression of 1 mmol (4·1 mg/100 ml).

  50 mmol sodium phosphate infused over 8 hours gives a mean serum Ca^{++} depression of 0·6 mmol (2·4 mg/100 ml).

  The only problem with using phosphate solution is the tendency to precipitate calcium salts out into the tissues. For this reason we would now suggest using either frusemide or mithramycin as first line therapy (*see* above).

(iv) If the patient has renal or cardiac failure, the volume of fluid and sodium load of this phosphate solution may be prohibitive and either mithramycin or dialysis (either peritoneal or haemo) against a calcium free dialysate should be undertaken.[26] As alternative to the above treatments, the following have been used.

(v) Calcitonin, whose role is still being evaluated,[24] but which can be used in a dose of 8 units/kg i.m. six-hourly, preferably as gelatin based porcine calcitonin;

(vi) if the situation is not critical, phosphate (Na_2HPO_4 or K_2HPO_4) 1–4 g/day may be given orally.

(4) As soon as the cause of the hypercalcaemia has been identified,[22] specific treatment should be started.

Tetany

DIAGNOSIS

(1) Is usually diagnosed by observing the characteristic carpo-pedal spasm of the hands (and sometimes feet). This is usually heralded by circumoral parasthesiae and may be accompanied by excessive neuromuscular irritability (the basis of Chvostek's sign).

(2) Is less easily recognised when it presents itself as laryngospasm, psychosis or generalised convulsions. Carpo-pedal spasm usually accompanies these manifestations, but if not, can usually be elicited by inflating a sphygmomanometer cuff above the systolic arterial pressure for 1 minute.

May be caused by:

(1) *Hypocalcaemia*. This occurs after parathyroid surgery, following a prolonged 'forced' diuresis, in malabsorbtion and in rickets and osteomalacia, sometimes immediately after vitamin D therapy is started. If it is unrelieved, pharyngeal spasm and generalised convulsions ensue. Psychotic behaviour may be prominent. Give 20 ml of 10% calcium gluconate i.v. over 10 minutes and continue with dihydrotachysterol—3–10 ml (0·25 mg/ml) per day initially but reducing rapidly. Monitor the serum Ca^{++} and PO_4^{--}.

(2) *Hyperventilation* (*see* p. 267).

(3) *Hypomagnasaemia*. This can also cause a positive Chvostek's sign and convulsions. Give 5–40 mmol magnesium sulphate or chloride slowly i.v. (1 mmol of magnesium chloride hexahydrate = 200 mg, 1 mmol of magnesium sulphate = 246 mg).

(4) *States of alkalotic hypokalaemia*. Usually seen when dehydration caused by vomiting is 'corrected' with infusions containing bicarbonate or lactate. Treatment is along the usual lines with potassium supplements, plus i.v. calcium gluconate as above.

(5) Rapid correction of chronic acidosis causes a decrease in ionised calcium and hence tetany. This is treated by giving calcium as in (1) above.

SECTION V REFERENCES

Hyperglycaemic coma

1   Aricff AI, Carroll HJ. Nonketotic hyperosmolar coma. *Medicine* (Baltimore) 1972; **51**: 73.

2   Clements RS, Blumenthal SA, Morrison AD, *et al.* Increased cerebro-spinal fluid pressure during treatment of diabetic ketoacidosis. *Lancet* 1971; **2**: 671.

3   Feig PU, McCuroy DK. The hypertonic state. *N Engl J Med* 1977; **297**: 1444.

4   Gerich JE, Martin MM, Recant L. Clinical and metabolic characteristics of hyperosmolar nonketotic coma. *Diabetes* 1971; **20**: 228.

5   Hockaday TDR, Alberti KGMM. Diabetic coma. *Br J Hosp Med* 1972; **7**: 183.

5a Leader. Treatment of severe hypophosphataemia. *Lancet* 1981; **2**: 734.

6   Joffe BI. Pathogenesis of nonketotic hyperosmolar diabetic coma. *Lancet* 1975; **1**: 1069.

7   Leader. Insulin regimes for diabetic ketoacidosis. *Br Med J* 1977; **1**: 405.

8   Page MMcB, Alberti KGMM, Greenwood R *et al.* Treatment of diabetic coma with continuous low dose infusion of insulin. *Br Med J* 1974; **2**: 687.

9   Thomas DJB, Gill B, Brown P, Stubbs WA. Salbutamol induced diabetic ketoacidosis. *Br Med J* 1977; **2**: 438.

Lactic acidosis

10 Alberti KGMM, Nattrass M. Lactic acidosis. *Lancet* 1977; **2**: 25.

11 Leader. Dichloro-acetate. *Br Med J* 1978; **2**: 456.

12 Relman AS. Lactic acidosis and a possible new treatment. *New Engl J Med* 1978; **298**: 564.

Hypoglycaemia

13 Jarrett RJ. Blood glucose homeostasis. *Br J Hosp Med* 1971; **6**: 499.

Hypopituitary coma

14 Garrod O. Hypopituitary coma. *Hospital Medicine* 1967; **2**: 300.

Thyroid

15 Evered D, Hall R. Hypothyroidism. *Br Med J* 1972; **1**: 290.

16 Herrman J, Ruddorff KH, Gockenjan G. Charcoal haemoperfusion in thyroid storm. *Lancet* 1977; **1**: 248.

17 Ikram H. Haemodynamic effects of beta-adrenergic blockade in hyperthyroid patients with and without heart failure. *Br Med J* 1977; **1**: 1505.

18 Mackin JF, Canary JJ, Pittmann CS. Thyroid storm and its management. *N Engl J Med* 1974; **291**: 1396.

19 Menedez CF, Rivilin RS. Thyrotoxic crisis and myxoedemic coma. *Med Clin Nth Am* 1973; **Nov**: 1463.

20 Perlmutter M. Myxoedema crisis of pituitary or thyroid origin. *Am J Med* 1964; **36**: 883.

21 Royce PC. Severely impaired consciousness in myxoedema. *Am J Med Sci* 1971; **261**: 46.

Acute hypercalcaemia and hypocalcaemia

22 Fraser P, Watson L, Healy M. Further experience with discriminant function in the differential diagnosis of hypercalcaemia. *Postgrad Med J* 1976; **52**: 254.

23 Fulmer DH, Dimich AB, Rothschild EO, *et al.* Treatment of hypercalcaemia. *Arch Intern Med* 1972; **129**: 923.

24 Leader. Treatment with calcitonin. *Br Med J* 1973; **1**: 1973.

25 Leader. Management of hypercalcaemic crisis. *Lancet* 1978; **2**: 617.

26 Nolph KD, Stoctz M, Maher JF. Calcium-free peritoneal dialysis. *Arch Intern Med* 1971; **128**: 809.

NEUROLOGICAL

The completed stroke[25]

DIAGNOSIS

This usually presents itself as a sudden neurological deficit in a person who may have pre-existing arterial disease. In addition there may be loss of consciousness.

(A) Strokes may be due to:

(1) *Cerebral infarction* (the majority). The vessels may be occluded by thrombosis *in situ*, or by embolic material arising from:

    (i)   *The heart*. Embolism is said to be rarely due to fibrillation alone unless the mitral valve is abnormal or the left atrium enlarged. Emboli arise from infected or calcified heart valves or from a prolapsing mitral valve.[9] Mural thrombi associated with myocardial infarction may become detached. Emboli from these sites may occlude vessels elsewhere and peripheral pulses must be checked.

    (ii)   *Neck vessels*. Commonly from atheromatous plaques at the origin of the internal carotid artery. A bruit may be heard but if stenosis is tight a bruit may be absent.

    (iii)   *Thrombosis* in situ. This usually occurs on atheromatous sections of the intra-cranial vessels. Thrombosis accounts for most internal capsular infarcts and also for most brain stem strokes, where occlusion of small end vessels causes ischaemic scars (lacunes). Lacunes[7] may cause a wide variety of syndromes but may recognisably present as:

        (a)   pure motor stroke;
        (b)   pure sensory stroke;
        (c)   dysarthria with a clumsy hand and;
        (d)   ipsilateral ataxia with weakness of the leg.

Cerebral infarction secondary to thrombosis is not always caused by atheromatous disease; and other causes such as arteritis (collagen disease), syphilis, the contraceptive pill[6] and polycythemia[26] should be excluded.

    In all forms of infarction, premonitory episodes of neurological deficit are not uncommon, meningism is rare, the CSF is not usually xanthochromic and unless there is massive infarction, there is no shift of midline structures within the first 24 hours. These features help to distinguish infarction from haemorrhage, a distinction which can be confirmed by a CT scan.

(2) *Cerebral haemorrhage* (the minority)[11]

(i) *Primarily intracerebral.* Bleeding in people with hypertension usually occurs from minute, thin-walled aneurysmal dilations of intracranial arteries—Charcot-Bouchard aneurysms. Occasionally, bleeding occurs from vascular malformations in normotensive patients. In about three-quarters of cases the bleeding spreads from the brain substance into the sub-arachnoid space and the resulting meningeal irritation gives rise to vomiting, headache and neck stiffness. Within the first 24 hours the haematoma, in about three-quarters of cases, causes a shift of midline structures (as identified by echoencephalography or by the position of the calcified pineal on an AP skull x-ray). CT scan reliably detects haemorrhage and, if this is readily available lumbar puncture should not be performed, because of the slight risk of coning. If CT scan is not available, an LP is still the best way of confirming haemorrhage.

(ii) *Primarily subarachnoid.*[17, 27] The bleeding occurs from an aneurysm or other malformation directly into the subarachnoid space. The symptoms, which characteristically start abruptly, are those of meningeal irritation, with or without loss of consciousness. Focal neurological deficits may be present due to arterial spasm or extension of haemorrhage into the brain. The combination of a focal neurological deficit in a patient with signs of sub-acute bacterial endocarditis strongly suggests mycotic aneurysm.[3] Blood in the subarachnoid space may be identified by CT scan and if so lumbar puncture is unnecessary. If the CT scan is unavailable or unrevealing, a lumbar puncture should be carried out—remember that occasionally an early LP will show normal CSF since it may take 24 hours for blood to appear in the lumbar CSF. All bloody CSF should be centrifuged so that subarachnoid bleeding identified by the xanthochromic supernatant, may be distinguished from a traumatic tap where the supernatant is clear. When a subarachnoid haemorrhage has been identified the timing of four vessel arteriography should be discussed with your neurosurgical colleagues.

(B) In any unconscious patient other causes of unconsciousness must be excluded (*see* p. 253).

In addition the following conditions may cause diagnostic confusion:

(1) *Subdural haematoma.* A history of head injury, while typical, may be lacking, especially in patients with pre-existing cortical atrophy. Percussion of the skull may reveal lateralised tenderness sufficient to arouse deeply stuporose patients, and also an area of dullness over the haematoma.[15]

Inequality of the pupils and a fluctuating but overall deteriorating level of consciousness, with progressive focal neurological signs are all highly suggestive.

There may be a shift of midline structures and the diagnosis may be confirmed with CT scan. However, if subdural haematomas are bilateral, there may be no mass effect, and if isodense, may be undetectable on CT scan. The very normality of the CT scan in a clearly deteriorating patient is in itself suspicious, and the diagnosis may be made by a radionucleide brain scan or if necessary arteriography.

(2) *Extra-dural haematoma.*

(3) *Brain tumour.* 3–5% of clinically diagnosed acute strokes turn out to be due to a tumour. Calcification may be present on skull x-ray or CT scan. Arteriography may reveal neovascularisation.

(4) *Brain abscess.* This usually occurs in the setting of purulent lung disease or in patients with a right to left intracardiac shunt. Ring enhancement is typically seen on CT scan but may be difficult to distinguish from a brain tumour.

(5) The differentiation from strokes of the mass lesions described in (1)–(4) above can only be made confidently with a CT scan. CT scans are not everywhere readily available, but in any 'stroke' patient who has a progression of their focal neurological deficit after you first see them, you should consider the desirability of obtaining a scan. We hope that as CT scans become more readily available, all 'salvageable' stroke patients will have one as part of the routine investigation.

(6) *Hemiplegic migraine.* A history of preceding or accompanying visual disturbance, a throbbing headache which is associated with nausea, and photophobia usually in a young person in association with a normal CSF clinches the diagnosis.

(7) Epileptic attacks, particularly those associated with residual paralysis (Todds paralysis) may also temporarily be mistaken for strokes.[16]

MANAGEMENT

The main purpose of the investigation is to determine if any treatable causes (*see* below), unfortunately the minority, are present. The history and clinical findings may help.

(1) The investigation of choice is a CT scan which may with a fair degree of reliability, demonstrate haemorrhage, subdural collections, abscess and tumour. It should be remembered, however, that the CT scan is not infallible and lesions, particularly of the brain stem and posterior fossa, can easily be missed.

(2) Radionucleide brain scans, particularly if 'dynamic' studies are incorporated, may provide more evidence of ischaemia than the CT scan. They may also demonstrate focal encephalitis, subdurals and other space occupying lesions.

(3) The skull x-ray still has a place and should be done particularly if there is any question of head injury.

(4) CSF examination may be undertaken if subarachnoid haemorrhage is suspected (*see* p. 166) but is of course contra-indicated in the presence of a space occupying lesion.

(5) Arteriography may be required to localise the space occupying lesion if a CT scan is not available, and is indicated in the further investigation of subarachnoid haemorrhage.

   Full blood picture and ESR, VDRL and FTA–ABS may detect the rare cases of collagen disease, syphilis, polycythemia, etc. which are treated on their merits.

(A) General measures

(1) General care of the helpless and/comatose patient (*see* p. 260).

(2) Treatment of complications which may follow a stroke.

   (i)   *Dehydration*. This is avoided by feeding fluids through a naso-gastric tube if the patient has a cough reflex, and if not, by giving fluids intravenously.

   (ii) *Hypothermia* (*see* p. 229).

   (iii) *Hyperthermia* (temperature $>40°C (104°F)$). This usually occurs in conjunction with a pontine lesion. If severe it may itself cause depression of consciousness; consequently, cooling the patient with tepid sponging is occasionally associated with marked improvement.

   (iv) *Diabetes*. This may be precipitated by an intracranial catastrophe. However, the transient glycosuria which may follow a stroke, needs no treatment unless ketosis occurs.

(v)   *Fits*. These need treatment in the usual way (*see* p. 182).

(vi)   *Hypertension*.[2] This may be a transient phenomenon, settl-
       ing within a few hours of the stroke. If it persists (i.e. a
       diastolic pressure above 120 mmHg) it would seem logical
       to reduce this to a level appropriate to the patient's age.
       However, following a stroke, the auto-regulatory capacity
       of blood vessels in the brain may be impaired for a period
       of about three weeks. This means that, in contradistinction
       to normal, the flow in the diseased area becomes pressure
       dependent, and so lowering arterial pressure will reduce
       flow to this area. Against this is the danger of continuing
       hypertension damaging the residual healthy brain. So we
       advocate, as a compromise, gentle reduction of arterial
       pressure until the diastolic is less than 110 mmHg and the
       systolic less than 170 mmHg. This should be accomplished
       where possible by conventional oral hypotensive therapy.
       Failing this, hydrallazine, initially 10 mg i.m. is a reason-
       able drug to use.

(vii) *Hypertensive encephalopathy*. The considerations in (vi)
       above do not apply if there is evidence of hypertensive
       encephalopathy (*see* p. 37).

(viii) *Cerebral oedema*. This may be seen as a mass effect on CT
       scan, and is occasionally manifest as papilloedema, and
       may reflect the volume of ischaemic tissue. There is no
       evidence that dexamethasone affects the oedema sur-
       rounding infarction or that it alters the mortality of mor-
       bidity following stroke. Dexamethasone is, however,
       extremely effective in reducing oedema surrounding
       tumour and abscess and may be given as 6 mg six-hourly.[3]
       However, if a stroke is sufficiently massive to threaten
       transtentorial herniation the outlook is necessarily poor
       and dexamethasone should be used with discretion. An
       acute rise in intracranial pressure may be treated by a
       bolus of 20% mannitol 1–2 g/kg i.v. over 5–10 minutes.
       Since a mannitol bolus may be followed by 'rebound'
       intracranial hypertension, infusion of 1 g/kg 20% man-
       nitol should be given over 8 hours subsequently.

(B) **Specific measures**

   In general determining the cause of a completed stroke has little
   immediate therapeutic spin-off. However, in the following situations specific therapy may be helpful.

(1) *Primary sub-arachnoid haemorrhage* (*see* above). There is real danger of re-bleeding in this group, and neurosurgical advice should be sought when the diagnosis is made. Treatment is likely to include an antifibrinolytic agent such as epsilon amino caproic acid (EACA) 24 g orally per day. Surgery to prevent re-bleeding may be of value in this group, particularly in the patient with little neurological impairment (*see* p. 166).

(2) *Cerebellar haematoma*. This merits separate mention as it is amenable to surgery. Unfortunately progression to coma and death is rapid due to brain stem compression. In the short interval before coma the patient may complain of occipital headache and vertigo. There is a gaze palsy to the side opposite the haemorrhage. Mild ipsilateral peripheral VIIth nerve palsy, dysarthria are common, but only a minority show nystagmus or ipsilateral ataxia. Contralateral hemiplegia does not occur, so the finding of a gaze palsy without limb paralysis is a useful pointer. Diagnosis is by CT scan or, failing that, arteriography.

(3) *Embolism*. The diagnosis of embolism rests on the acute onset of neurological deficit in a patient with a source of emboli, e.g. atrial fibrillation. Further emboli may be prevented by adequate anticoagulation. However, 30% of infarcts secondary to embolism are haemorrhagic as demonstrated on CT scan or by the presence of blood or xanthochromia in the cerebrospinal fluid. Early anticoagulation in this group may precipitate disastrous secondary haemorrhage and should be delayed for approximately two weeks. It follows from the above that it is highly desirable to get a CT scan before starting a course of anticoagulants.

(4) When any of the causes considered under differential diagnosis are found, appropriate therapy should be instituted.

Transient ischaemic attacks (TIA)[10,19,21]

DIAGNOSIS

These are episodes of transient neurological deficit. They may be recurrent, sometimes only last a few minutes, and are usually due to temporary reduction in blood supply to part of the brain. The importance of recognising TIA's is that they are followed by major stroke with a frequency of about 5% per annum.

They may be caused by:

(1) Emboli arising from atheroma of the vertebral and carotid arteries, or their branches, or from the heart.
(2) In the setting of borderline local cerebral perfusion, transient reduction in overall cerebral blood flow may cause significant but temporary local ischaemia. This can occur on the basis of:

    (i)   A fall in perfusion pressure due to:

        (a) Hypotension (e.g. hypotensive drugs (*see* p. 38);
        (b) Decreased cardiac output (e.g. arrhythmias).[12]

    (ii)   Increased viscosity:

        (a) A PCV of above 50%;[25]
        (b) Paraproteinaemia.

(3) Transient reduction in local blood flow:

    (i)   Hypertension. Focal neurological deficit may occur as part of hypertensive encephalopathy (*see* p. 37).
    (ii)   Migraine. Complicated migraine may occasionally cause hemiplegia characterised more by dysasthesiae than weakness, or a third or sixth nerve palsy (ophthalmoplegic migraine). It is usually possible to elicit a history of previous attacks of 'classical' migraine.
    (iii) Mechanical effects on flow.

        (a) Neck movements may cause occlusion of the vertebral arteries with ensuing posterior cerebral and brain stem ischaemia. Failure of autoregulation of the posterior cerebral circulation may cause the structures so supplied to be vulnerable to changes of the systemic circulation. This may play a role in 'vertebral basilar insufficiency'.[22]

(b) Similarly carotid arteries may also be occluded by neck movements particularly if they are kinked or tortuous.

(c) Subclavian steal. In this condition movement of the arms diverts blood from the vertebral arteries causing symptoms of transient brain stem ischaemia.

(4) Lack of nutrients:

(i) *Anaemia*. Haemoglobin of less than 7 g/100 ml may be the sole cause of TIA.

(ii) *Hypoglycaemia*. This may rarely present itself with a focal neurological deficit presumably on the same basis as in (2) above.

In a proportion of cases no cause can be found presumably because of lysis of the vascular obstruction, or because the vessel involved is too small to be identified.

(5) TIAs should be differentiated from:

(i) Focal epilepsy. In focal epilepsy, the patient often complains of positive symptoms (e.g. paraethesiae, spontaneous movements). These are uncommon in TIAs.

(ii) Todd's paralysis.

(6) Attacks resembling TIAs may be the initial symptoms of cerebral tumours. These are presumably caused by alteration of circulation in the adjacent brain.

Examination therefore must include careful auscultation of the head, heart and neck, measurement of lying and standing arterial pressure and the pressure in each arm and assessment of peripheral vasculature. A 24-hour continuous ECG, plasma glucose, lipid profile and cholesterol and full blood picture may establish an underlying cause which should be dealt with accordingly. A prolapsing leaflet of the mitral valve may give rise to a loud mid-systolic click or be silent. It can however, be detected by echocardiography.[9] Non-invasive investigation has been discussed elsewhere.[1]

MANAGEMENT

There are several uncontroversial aspects of management.
  These include:

(1) Control of hypertension.[2] The diastolic pressure should be slowly reduced to less than 100 mmHg. Thiazide diuretics and propranolol are useful hypotensive agents as they minimise the chances of postural hypotension. Reduction of arterial pressure may be all that is required to control TIA.
(2) Control of blood glucose.
(3) Reduction of PCV to below 45% by repeated small (200 cc) venesections.[20]
(4) Reduction of hypercholesterolaemia or hyperlipidaemia.
(5) Prophylactic anticoagulants following emboli arising from the heart.

Three other modes of therapy each have their proponents:

(1) Endarterectomy.[24, 25]
(2) Prophylactic anticoagulants.
(3) Inhibition of platelet function with aspirin 150 mg daily or sulfinpyrazone 200 mg q.d.s.

It is possible that TIAs due to atheromatous disease of the cerebral blood vessels have several causes, and that different subgroups of patients are affected (favourably or adversely) by these methods of treatment. Well-controlled trials of each against no treatment are rare and against each other are non-existent. In our current ignorance one accepted course of practice is to perform four vessel arteriography in patients who are otherwise surgically acceptable and in whom no other cause has been found (*see* above) and to operate on significant stenosis or deeply ulcerated plaques.

  Anticoagulants may be used in patients with intrinsic carotid disease where no operable lesion is identified, who have no medical contraindication, who are judged to take medicines reliably, and who can be closely supervised. Aspirin and sulfinpyrazone may be used in the remainder. It should be remembered, however, that the major cause of death in patients with TIAs, is cardiovascular disease and that treatment directed solely to the cerebral circulation may be irrelevant to the patient as a whole.

Closed head injury

DIAGNOSIS

(1) Is not usually in doubt, but needs to be considered with every unconscious patient and witnesses should be sought.

(2) Can usually be made following careful examination of the head and neck. Blood and/or CSF in the external auditory canal or behind the tympanic membrane indicates a basal skull fracture. An anterior fossa fracture may be indicated by CSF rhinorrhoea or periorbital haematomata. Vitreous haemorrhage may occur following a whiplash injury, particularly in children.

(3) May occur in the setting of other conditions some of which may also cause coma—for example, acute alcoholic intoxication. In this situation, as in all situations of suspected head injury, the skull should be x-rayed. A skull fracture cannot be diagnosed clinically, is a strong indication of the severity of the injury and may therefore be associated with intracranial pathology which may only become apparent after an interval.

(4) Consideration should be given to injury elsewhere—particularly the neck (*see* below on p. 175).

MANAGEMENT

Head injuries may give rise to unconsciousness and death because of the contusion and haemorrhage sustained at the time. Frequently however it is events subsequent to the injury which account for considerable morbidity and mortality. The major part of this is the development of cerebral oedema, which in turn compromises cerebral blood flow. In addition, other reversible factors include hypoxia, hypotension usually secondary to hypovolaemia, fits and infection. Due attention must be given to these secondary events which do not themselves require special neurosurgical expertise, but are at least as important as the consequences of the primary injury.

In rough order of priority therefore:

(1) Check the airway. If ventilation is in doubt either because of brain stem involvement or for peripheral reasons (inhaled blood or vomit or chest injury) intubate and ventilate.

(2) Check the arterial pressure. Hypotension usually results from blood loss from injuries elsewhere but occurs occasionally for central reasons. Treatment is along the usual lines with volume (usually blood) replacement and pressor agents if necessary (*see* p. 245).

(3) Control fits—if any (p. 182).

(4) Examine the neck. If there is local pain, evidence of trauma or evidence of loss of power or sensation in the limbs do not move the patient until a lateral neck x-ray has been obtained.

(5) Do not give opiates for pain, phenobarbitone for restlessness or mydriatics for convenient observation of the fundi since interpretation of the pupillary response is extremely important.

(6) When the ventilation, circulation and fits are satisfactorily controlled, assess the level of consciousness. We recommend the use of the Glasgow coma scale. Three elements of behaviour are scored:

(i) *Eye opening.*

Response	Score	
Nil	1	(no response to any stimulus)
Pain	2	(infra-orbital pressure)
Verbal	3	(response to a loud command)
Spontaneous	4	

(ii) *Motor response (to infra-orbital pressure).*

Response	Score	
Nil	1	
Abnormal extension	2	(extension of both arms and legs)
Abnormal flexion	3	(flexion preceded by extension)
Weak flexion	4	(flexor withdrawal response)
Localising	5	(able to use a limb to locate and resists the noxious stimulus)
Obeys commands	6	

(The arms are usually more responsive than the legs; in the case of different patterns in arms and legs, always record the *best* response.)

(iii) *Verbal response*

Response	Score
Nil	1

Response	Score	
Incomprehensible	2	(mumbling—no recognisable words)
Inappropriate	3	(intelligible, isolated words—often profanities—no phrases)
Confused	4	(correct phrases, but disorientated and confused in context)
Fully orientated	5	

Information derived from these observations should be recorded on a chart. Deterioration in the level of consciousness implies progression of the neuronal damage. This calls for an urgent re-appraisal of the situation usually by a more experienced colleague.

Patients with significant head injuries fall into one of three groups:

(A) *Spontaneous improvement* (the majority). These patients need careful observation in hospital and, if all is well, can usually be discharged 24 hours after they have fully recovered. Careful observation should consist for at least 6 hours of quarter-hourly recording and charting of:

(i)   Pulse;
(ii) Arterial pressure.

Charting of these allows the trend to be recognised if the pulse is slowing or arterial pressure rising in the case of increasing intracranial pressure; similarly a rising pulse and falling arterial pressure will indicate occult haemorrhage.

(iii) Respiration. An altered ventilatory pattern (and/or depth) may indicate brain stem compromise (p. 256).
(iv) Conscious level (*see* above).
(v)   Pupillary size and reactivity. Ipsilateral constriction followed by dilatation of a pupil on the side of the subdural or extradural haematoma occurs, but only in the minority. Increasingly large and sluggish pupils warn of a general increase in intracranial pressure (but rarely without increasing drowsiness and perhaps vomiting also).

(B) *Deteriorating conscious level* (with or without localising neurological signs). Examination of the patient even in coma can be surprisingly complete. Particular attention should be paid to brain stem reflexes since these may have the greater prognostic significance (p. 255). In addition to lateralised weakness, sensory loss and asymmetrical deep tendon reflexes should be looked for. Deterioration may be due either to the development of cerebral oedema or haematoma. Both may be fatal or cause secondary morbidity. Both need urgent treatment, haematomas sub- or extradural by exploration. If the patient is deteriorating rapidly or you do not have a CT scanner on site you should proceed to theatres without delay. Following this, or if this degree of haste is not indicated, a CT scan is of great help in management indicating the presence of blood or brain swelling secondary to oedema. The effective control of cerebral oedema should reduce secondary morbidity or mortality.

This is achieved by:

(i)   Hyperventilation. The patient should be paralysed and ventilated to achieve a Paco$_2$ of 25–30 mmHg. This is best achieved by an initial dose of pancuronium bromide (Pavulon) of 50–100 μg/kg i.v. and followed at 1–1·5 hourly intervals by further doses of 60 μg/kg i.v. or i.m.
(ii) 20% mannitol 1·5 g/kg i.v. infused over 10 minutes.
(iii) Dexamethasone 0·5 mg/kg/day given six-hourly.

Following the institution of these measures, arrangements should be made for continuous monitoring of intracranial pressure by, for example, a subdural catheter.

If a general anaesthetic is necessary, ketamine and halothane, both of which may raise the intracranial pressure, should be avoided.

If the intracranial pressure is found to be normal, no further mannitol need be given and the hyperventilation can be reduced progressively over a 24-hour period. If the intracranial pressure recurs, then hyperventilation is obviously reinstituted.

If the pressure remains elevated at more than 20 mmHg despite the above, barbiturate narcosis is worth trying. Pentobarbitone 20 mg/kg is given as a loading dose and followed by 4 mg/kg doses to maintain the serum level between 30–40 μg/l (132·6–176·8 mmol/l).

However, dexamethasone and hyperventilation alone may control the intracranial pressure adequately for 90% of the time with occasional apparently 'spontaneous' rises to 40 mmHg or more. Some of these spontaneous rises may be triggered by the lack of sedation, increasing $Pa\text{co}_2$ (more than 30 mmHg) or hypoxaemia (less than 85 mmHg). These causes should be looked for and in any case a 1·5 g/kg bolus of mannitol given as above. The effect of this lasts for about 4 hours. If further mannitol is necessary a temporising measure is to give this dose as a 4-hour infusion. The serum osmolality should be checked and not allowed to rise above 325 mosmol/kg. If, despite this, the intracranial pressure rises above 20 mmHg barbiturate narcosis should be started as above.

(C) *Initial deep coma.* No eye opening, no verbal response to pain and either no motor response or abnormal flexion ('decorticate') or extension ('decerebrate') of the arms (Glasgow coma scale of 5 or less). The treatment is exclusion of an intracranial haematoma and control of intracranial pressure as above, but the group is here distinguished because the prognosis is worse.

If, despite the above, the intracranial pressure remains uncontrolled, two further measures have been advocated:

(i) Hypothermia. Whilst this may reduce the brain's metabolic demands, we are unconvinced that it has any practical beneficial effect.
(ii) Extensive craniotomy.

However, if either of these steps have to be contemplated, the patient is in a high mortality group with, in the event of survival, almost inevitable major handicap. A case can be made, therefore, for withdrawal of life support at this point.

(7) The aim of management is to maintain a cerebral perfusion pressure of at least 60 mmHg. The cerebral perfusion pressure is the mean arterial pressure minus the intracranial pressure. The mean arterial pressure is roughly: diastolic pressure + (systolic pressure − diastolic pressure)/3. If, therefore, the circulation needs support, this defines the level you should be aiming at.
(8) Fits should be treated with phenytoin (p. 182).
(9) Antibiotics should be given:

(i) If there is CSF or blood dripping from the ear or nose. CSF from the nose can be differentiated from mucus as only the former contains glucose (use a BM stix).

(ii) If the skull x-ray shows a fracture running into a sinus or the middle ear or the presence of intracranial air.

(iii) Evidence of a basilar or anterior fossa fracture (*see* above).

(iv) Significantly (more than 5 mm) depressed fractures.

Since pneumococcus is the most likely organism to cause meningitis secondary to head trauma, penicillin 15–20 mega units/day i.v. divided into four-hourly doses should be given until the CSF leak is stopped, the depressed fracture is elevated, or 5 days, whichever is the longer.

(10) Other complications which you need to be alert for include:

(i) Hyperpyrexia. Sponging, fanning and antipyretics including chlorpromazine are the mainstays of treatment.

(ii) Inappropriate ADH secretion. The resulting hyponatraemia nearly always responds to fluid restriction and replacement of insensible fluid loss with normal saline.

FURTHER READING

Jennet B, Teasdale G. *Management of head injuries*. Contemporary Neurology Series. Philadelphia: F.A. Davis Co., 1981.

Jeffreys RV, Jones JJ. Avoidable factors contributing to the death of head injury patients in general hospitals. *Lancet* 1981; **2**: 459.

Faints

DIAGNOSIS

Fainting is usually defined as a transient loss of consciousness due to cerebral ischaemia, caused in turn by a reduction in blood supply to the brain. The commonest type is the so-called simple faint. This occurs for example in young girls at school assemblies, who have gone without breakfast, or in elderly patients who get up after a period of bed rest. It is said to be due to blood pooling in the leg veins. It is more likely to occur in people who are anaemic, tired or frightened, or who are easily affected by the sight of blood or other people fainting.

(1) However, a few faints are caused by serious underlying disease:

    (i)   any stenoic heart valve lesion;

    (ii)   constrictive pericarditis;

    (iii) cardiac arrhythmias (especially ventricular tachycardia and Stokes-Adams attacks);

    (iv) myocardial infarction;

    (v)   a severe haemorrhage;

    (vi) involvement of the autonomic nervous system with hypotensive agents, diabetes, syringomyelia, tabes dorsalis and other rarer causes of autonomic neuropathy;

    (vii) vertebrobasilar insufficiency—in patients with cervical spondylosis, turning of the head may cause spurs of bone to occlude the vertebral artery (but also *see* p. 171).

    (viii) any cause of severe pain;

    (ix) rarely a subclavian 'steal'.

(2) A few more are provoked by relatively benign stimuli:

    (i)   micturition syncope;

    (ii)   cough and laugh syncope;

    (iii) carotid sinus syncope;

    (iv) venepuncture and pleural puncture.

(3) Cerebral ischaemia is one of the many triggers for a convulsion. Faints, therefore, if prolonged can cause fits. Such patients should not be considered to have epilepsy.

(4) Some other conditions which cause transient alteration of consciousness include:

    (i)   transient ischaemic attacks (TIA) (*see* p. 171);
    (ii)   epilepsy (*see* p. 182);
    (iii)   severe hypertension (*see* p. 37)—remember that transient losses of consciousness may be due to sudden elevation, as well as sudden drops, in arterial pressure;
    (iv)   hypotension (*see* p. 241).
    (v)   hyperventilation (*see* p. 267);
    (vi)   cataplexy;
    (vii) paroxysmal vertigo.

MANAGEMENT

All that needs to be done in the simple faint is to lie the patient flat, or with head slightly down, relieve any compression of the neck and maintain an airway. As indicated above, a careful history and full examination is mandatory if serious conditions are not to be missed.

Fits[33]

The common grand mal convulsion is usually self limiting. All that is required is to see that the patient has an airway (turn the patient on his side and remove false teeth), does not bang against furniture or roll into the fire. The patient should not be actively restrained and well meaning attempts to depress the tongue are unnecessary and frequently traumatic.

Repeated tonic clonic seizures without recovery between attacks or one seizure lasting more than 30 minutes—status epilepticus—is an emergency because irreversible brain damage may occur. This occurs on the basis of hypoxia, hyperpyrexia, and hypotension as well as continuing electrical activity which itself may cause neuronal damage.[32]

MANAGEMENT

(1) Suppressing the fits is the first priority.

    (i)   The drug of choice is one of the benzodiazepines.[29, 30] Give either clonazepam 1–2 mg i.v. or diazepam 10 mg i.v. Repeat the dose if seizure activity has not ceased within 5 minutes. Since diazepam precipitates when diluted, slow infusions should not be used. The same strictures probably apply to clonazepam.

Benzodiazepines can produce respiratory depression, particularly if your patient has had a recent dose of another anticonvulsant drug.

    (ii)   If the benzodiazepines fail to control the fits, phenytoin sodium should be used. Infuse 15–20 mg/kg of ready-made infusion fluid—250 mg/5 ml over 45 minutes. This drug has the advantage of not impairing the conscious level and thus allowing an early neurological assessment. Phenytoin sodium must not be added to any other i.v. infusion as an acid precipitate may form. In the unlikely event that seizures are not controlled by the above measures, alternatives include:

(iii)   Chlormethiazole.[31] Use 500 ml of an 0·8% solution over 6–8 hours. This drug may also cause hypotension and respiratory depression.

(iv)   Amylobarbitone 3–5 mg/kg i.v. at a rate not greater than 100 mg/min. This drug may rarely cause laryngospasm, depresses the conscious level and also depresses respiration.

    Amylobarbital should only be used when facilities for assisted ventilation are readily available.

(v)   Intramuscular paraldehyde 5 ml into each buttock is still an occasional useful standby particularly if intravenous drugs cannot be used. Since it is painful its use should be avoided unless the patient is unconscious. It is generally given using glass syringes since it is said to dissolve plastic. In practice it is safe to use modern plastic syringes provided it is given immediately. For practical purposes it does not cause respiratory depression.

(vi)   As a last resort, you may have to paralyse the patient.[28] In these circumstances your best guide to successful therapy is some form of EEG (the single channel recording of a cerebral function monitor is sufficient). This will tell you when you have succeeded in controlling the abnormal electrical activity, which you must do, as this continuing activity may itself cause brain damage.

(2) Determining the cause.

(i)   In patients with epilepsy, status may be caused by either a deficiency or an excess of their anticonvulsants. Always do urgent anticonvulsant blood levels to determine the patient's drug status.

(ii)   If status is the first manifestation of seizures, acute progressive disease is usually responsible. Unless papilloedema is present, lumbar puncture should be performed to look for meningitis. In the presence of papilloedema the procedures to define an intracranial space occupying lesion are, in order of preference, computerised tomography, radio-nucleide brain scan or four vessel arteriography.

(iii)   Hypoglycaemia, hypocalcaemia and hypoxia may provoke seizures. Do a BM stix, blood glucose, plasma calcium and arterial blood gases.

(3) After the fits have been controlled.

(i)   Examine the patient including his mouth carefully as injuries during the fits are common.

(ii)   Then allow the sleep which occurs after fits to continue.

(iii) Initiate maintenance therapy with one of the major anti-convulsants, phenobarbitone, carbamazepine or pheny-toin. I.V. phenytoin may be given as a loading dose as above (never give it by i.m. injection as it is absorbed erratically).

Spinal cord compression

DIAGNOSIS

(1) May be suggested by a history of paraparesis associated with paraesthesiae or root pain brought on or exacerbated by movement. Physical examination may establish a sensory motor, sweating or reflex level which is a guide to the level of compression.

(2) Sudden cord lesions in the absence of trauma, may be caused by either intramedullary or extramedullary pathology.

Whilst the attempt to distinguish the two is an interesting clinical exercise, the conclusions are frequently wrong particularly when the onset of symptoms is acute. The distinction is made by myelography which should be performed as soon as possible (*see* below). Clinical points we have found useful include:

(i) well localised spinal tenderness as revealed by percussion suggests epidural abscess;

(ii) previous and remote neurological episodes, e.g. retrobulbar neuritis, suggests demyelinating disease;

(iii) a previous and ill advised lumbar puncture performed in a patient with deranged coagulation suggests extradural haematoma;

(iv) extradural tumours are most commonly metastases from elsewhere and extraspinal primaries should always be looked for.

MANAGEMENT

Cord compression sufficient to cause symptoms and signs for more than a few hours causes irreversible cord damage. Your neurosurgical colleagues should be consulted as soon as the diagnosis is suspected and investigations carried out in conjunction with them. The next priority is to obtain spinal x-ray films which may reveal erosion of pedicles or vertebral bodies suggesting extradural lesions, followed by myelography. If the technique is available this is most safely performed above the block by a C1-2 puncture.

Acute ascending polyneuritis[34,35]

DIAGNOSIS

(1) Is made from a characteristic history of onset of weakness which involves first the legs then the arms and may spread to involve the bulbar muscles, face and respiratory muscles. This often starts five to twelve days after a mild virus infection. Commonly, weakness may be preceded by paraesthesiae and mild sensory loss. Sometimes muscle tenderness is also present. Deep tendon reflexes are absent.

(2) Differentiation is from other causes of acute weakness:

    (i) Acute poliomyelitis. The paralysis which is nearly always asymmetrical and confined within muscle groups is generally preceded by mild meningitic symptoms by three to four days. In addition, sensory signs are never found in 'polio'.

    (ii) Tick paralysis is an important consideration in some countries, including the US and Australia. The less accessible parts of the anatomy should be carefully searched since removal of the offending tick is followed by dramatic return of power.

    (iii) Other causes of acute polyneuritis, e.g. porphyria and diphtheria, are distinguished by examination or simple tests. Botulism also causes generalised weakness but the onset is typically bulbar, and characteristically associated with severe constipation.

(3) Cerebrospinal fluid usually contains a raised protein and normal cell count at some stage of the illness but may be normal initially. A urine VMA should always be performed in children because of the association with neuroblastoma. Nerve conduction velocities are significantly slowed at least in some portions of the nerves (since this is a disease of segmental demyelination) in all cases.

MANAGEMENT

(1) There is no specific treatment. The incidence of subsequent relapse is actually greater if steroids have been used. In a recent

186

well controlled trial, plasmaphaeresis was shown to speed recovery, and may prove to be an effective therapy.[35] Management is entirely supportive and artificial ventilation is indicated urgently if paralysis of intercostal muscles or the diaphragm occurs.

(2) The power of the respiratory muscles may be assessed clinically in the first instance by asking the patient to count in exhalation. The patient takes a maximal inspiration, and begins to count off seconds from a clock until he is forced to take another breath. Power is impaired if the patient cannot go beyond 15 seconds. Whilst respiration is jeopardised this test should be performed hourly.

(3) As always, however, the best measures of the efficiency of ventilation is the level of the blood gases and simple respiratory function tests. If respiration is compromised the blood gases should be done regularly (at least six-hourly) and the vital capacity measured two-hourly with a spirometer.

(4) Artificial ventilation must be used if CO_2 retention ($Paco_2$ more than 45 mmHg) and hypoxia (Pao_2 less than 75 mmHg) occur. This becomes necessary in about a quarter of all patients between 2 to 21 days from the onset of symptoms.

(5) Respiratory failure can occur very rapidly with little previous distress or deterioration in the counting ability or the blood gases. Equipment for endo-tracheal intubation should be at hand—together with a ventilator (preferably out of sight).

(6) Respiratory embarrassment may also occur if bulbar paralysis is unrecognised. Nasal secretions and saliva accumulate in the pharynx, and intubation followed by tracheostomy with a cuffed tube may be required in order to protect the airway.

(7) Autonomic disturbances, such as spontaneous fluctuation of the blood pressure and pulse rate may occur—yet another reason for the meticulous monitoring required in these patients. Propranolol 40 mg b.d. (if necessary via a naso-gastric tube) will usually control these autonomic problems.

(8) Full recovery of muscular function often occurs after total paralysis. The main factor influencing survival is meticulous and full nursing care with special attention to tracheostomy toilet, prevention of bed sores, muscle contractures, wrist and foot drop and evacuation of bowels and bladder. Loss of sphincter control is common, and regular suppositories and an in-dwelling bladder catheter may be necessary.

Details of management of the totally paralysed patient are beyond the scope of this book.

Myasthenia gravis[37,39]

DIAGNOSIS

(1) Is made from a history of characteristic fatigue on continued exertion. In mild cases, power is normal after a period of rest, but then declines abnormally quickly on exercise. In more severe cases weakness is constant. The weakness may be generalised or confined to particular groups of muscles, e.g. the extra-ocular muscles or bulbar muscles. The onset of easy fatiguability is usually insidious—occurring only at the end of the day—but occasionally it is acute. Fatiguability is demonstrated by continued use of specific muscles for a short period of time. There is no sensory loss and the reflexes are nearly always preserved.

(2) The diagnosis is confirmed by the Tensilon test. Decide which muscle groups are weakest. Choose the three most evident and also measure the forced vital capacity (FVC). Give edrophonium (Tensilon) 2 mg i.v. stat and if there is no sweating, salivation, lacrimation, colic or muscle fasciculation during the next minute give a further 8 mg i.v. If these unpleasant cholinergic side-effects do occur they may be aborted by atropine 1·0 mg i.v. Re-assess the three muscle groups and re-measure the FVC within the next minute. Frequently the response is equivocal—some muscle groups responding dramatically and others not at all. If the overall response is indecisive repeat the test later in the day and try to gauge the general trend. If there is still genuine doubt, the effect of Tensilon on the motor response to repetitive nerve stimulation can be studied.

(3) Differentiation is from other causes of weakness.

MANAGEMENT

(1) Start prednisone in high dose, e.g. 80 mg daily. Most authorities would also prepare the patient for thymectomy. During the first two weeks of steroid therapy increasing fatiguability may be evident. Thus, for these first 2 weeks the patient must remain in hospital.

(2) During this period pyridostigmine (Mestinon) 60–180 mg every six hours may be necessary, the dose being adjusted to provide maximum response without side effects. Oral, subcutaneous, and intra-muscular preparations are available as necessary.

(3) Thereafter it is usually possible to taper the Mestinon and maintain the patient on a slowly reducing alternate-day steroid regimen.

MYASTHENIC CRISIS
(Too Little Treatment)

DIAGNOSIS

The myasthenic crisis is an exacerbation of weakness which most often occurs in an already diagnosed myasthenic patient. It is less frequent than formerly, now that treatment regimes are based on immunosuppression rather than anticholinesterases. However, it may occur in a previously undiagnosed patient and be precipitated by stress, emotion, infection or trauma, or by drugs which block neuromuscular transmission, e.g. streptomycin, gentamicin, kanamycin, lincomycin, and colomycin. Anaesthetists are fully conversant with the prolonged action of suxamethonium in these patients.

MANAGEMENT

Give edrophonium (Tensilon) as outlined above (see p. 188). An immediate improvement in muscle power indicates that the patient requires further anticholinesterase therapy, in addition to the immunosuppressive therapy he may already be receiving. Therefore, proceed as outlined for management of myasthenia. While pyridostigmine is taking effect it may be necessary to support respiration on a ventilator. Occasionally severe weakness requiring ventilatory support persists despite full immunosuppression. In this situation plasmapheresis may be life saving.[39]

CHOLINERGIC CRISIS
(Too Much Treatment)

DIAGNOSIS

(1) Is precipitated by excessive anticholinesterases. It occurs within half an hour to two hours after the previous dose, typically at the time when steroid therapy is beginning to take effect.

(2) The initial warning symptoms and signs are colic, sweating, salivation and fasciculation. These symptoms are sufficiently clear and drug related for it to be extremely rare for further progression to develop. However, deliberate over-administration may proceed via nervousness, drowsiness and confusion to ataxia, dysarthria, hypertension and bradycardia culminating in coma, which may be interrupted by convulsions, and finally death. The warning signs may be masked if atropine or atropine-like drugs are given with the anticholinesterases. Helpful physical signs may be small pupils (less than 3 mm in diameter) and fasciculation which persists to a late stage.

(3) It is obviously crucial to distinguish this from a myasthenic crisis, which is the commonest cause of acute weakness in a myasthenic patient. If there is still doubt after the history and examination give edrophonium (Tensilon) 10 mg i.v. with a ventilator at hand. If there is improvement, the weakness is due to a myasthenic crisis. If there is no response or a deterioration the diagnosis is a cholinergic crisis.

MANAGEMENT

(1) Stop pyridostigmine.

(2) Give atropine sulphate 1 mg i.v. half-hourly to a maximum of 8 mg.

(3) Maintain respiration. If acute respiratory failure occurs the patient is ventilated in the usual way. If acute respiratory failure has not occurred the power of the respiratory muscles may be assessed clinically by having the patient count in exhalation and perform other simple respiratory function tests (*see* p. 187). This should be done hourly. In addition the blood gases should be measured regularly (the $Paco_2$ should be checked at least six-

hourly) and should also be done immediately if any deterioration of the counting test occurs.

(4) Reformation of cholinesterase should be assessed by response to the edrophonium test, which should be performed two-hourly until temporary return of muscle power occurs. At this point a small dose of oral pyridostigmine (e.g. 30 mg) should be tried.

Generalised tetanus[41]

DIAGNOSIS

(1) The typical case is entirely characteristic and quite unforgett-able. The history is of dysphagia and stiffness and pain in the muscles of the neck, back and abdominal wall. Examination reveals hypertonia, usually greater in the extended legs than in the arms, together with painless trismus. In all but the milder cases the rigid posture is interrupted by paroxysms in which extension of the back, neck and legs and flexion of the shoulders and elbows is accompanied by the characteristic grimaces. These last up to 20 seconds and are painful. Rigidity persists between paroxysms, thus distinguishing tetanus from strychnine poison-ing and rabies.

If the time between the onset of rigidity and the onset of spasms is no more than a few hours, subsequent paroxysms are likely to be frequent and to occur for several days.

(2) The attack may be modified by previous immunisation—the spasm remaining localised to the site of infection.

(3) The site of entry should be sought. Apart from obvious puncture wounds and infected umbilical stumps, this includes ruptured tympanic membranes usually associated with an ear discharge.

Before treatment is instituted the patient should be watched for a period of 10–15 minutes while he is lying relaxed in a quiet and darkened room. The extent of rigidity and the number of spasms which occur during this period provide a baseline upon which the effects of treatment may be assessed.

MANAGEMENT

Involves:

(1) Suppressing the organism and its toxin.

    (i)   Give Human Tetanus Immunoglobin (Humotet 100 i.u./kg intramuscularly (never intravenously)—a previous test dose being unnecessary). In the event of unavailability of human immunoglobulins, you should still give the

192

heterologous anti-tetanus serum (ATS). Give 0·2 ml as a test dose, and if there is no reaction within half an hour, give 5000 units of ATS i.m. Intrathecal Human Tetanus Immunoglobulin has been shown to be of benefit if given in early tetanus. The dose is 250 i.u. instilled intrathecally.[42]

(ii) Give benzyl penicillin 1 mega unit six-hourly.

(iii) Excise all dead tissues surrounding the wound (if any) not less than one hour after the patient has been protected by ATS and penicillin. The wound is kept open and irrigated with hydrogen peroxide or 1 × 4000 potassium permanganate solution three times a day.

(2) Treating rigidity—if the patient is developing rigidity start with chlorpromazine 75 mg four-hourly orally. If this does not prove effective, add sodium amytal 150 mg orally six-hourly between injections of chlorpromazine. The aim is to achieve a state of light sleep for most of the time. If this regime is ineffective add diazepam 10 mg orally every 4 hours or meprobamate 400 mg orally every 4 hours. Remember that patients with rigidity have increased fluid and calorie requirements. If these drugs in combination do not produce relaxation curarisation and artificial ventilation (IPPR) are indicated (*see* below).

(3) Treating spasms—spasms are painful and dangerous as they may cause hypoxia and crush fractures of the spine and must be controlled by curarisation and IPPR. Spasms occur in response to a stimulus. This may be a distended bladder, faecal impaction or bronchial mucus and effective control of spasms may be secured by eliminating these stimuli rather than by increasing the dose of drugs.

Swallowing also may precipitate spasms. For this reason, if the disease is likely to be severe (short period of onset) a naso-gastric tube should be passed early rather than late. Nursing attention must be kept to an absolute minimum. The single spasms which need to be treated urgently—for example, laryngospasm—may respond to chlorpromazine 100 mg i.v.

(4) Curarisation and IPPR are indicated:

(i) If rigidity is uncontrolled and makes breathing difficult.

(ii) If laryngospasm occurs. This is an absolute indication. Laryngospasm may be precipitated by attempts to pass a naso-gastric or endo-tracheal tube and these procedures should not be attempted in the interval between the first episode of laryngospasm and the ensuing tracheostomy.

(iii)   In every patient who has generalised spasm.

Complete muscle relaxation and IPPR may necessitate transfer to a specialised unit, for the chances of a successful outcome depend largely on meticulous and intensive nursing care which may be necessary for 6 weeks or more. To the usual hazards of this sort of treatment are added other more specific complications to which patients with tetanus are especially liable, e.g. hyperpyrexia and bacterial shock, autonomic imbalance and arrhythmias.[40]

Brain death

The advent of prolonged ventilation has given rise to a group of patients with brain death. The non-functioning brain stem is followed, usually within a few days, by asystole *despite* continued ventilation. Thus, given certain vital pre-requisites, a non-functioning brain stem can be regarded as an alternative form of death—brain death.

This is an important diagnosis for two reasons:

(1) It allows organ donation to proceed.
(2) It allows ventilation to be discontinued.

The diagnosis of brain death cannot be considered until certain conditions have been excluded:

(1) Intoxication with narcotics, hypnotics or tranquillisers. This entails a specific enquiry and full drug screen. Since there is insufficient knowledge about the effects of therapeutic concentrations of phenobarbitone (when used as an anticonvulsant) when associated with brain injury, the assessment of brain stem function for the diagnosis of brain death should be deferred until blood levels of phenobarbitone are extremely low.
(2) Hypothermia. The core (rectal) temperature should be not less than 35°C.
(3) Action of relaxants—neuromuscular blocking agents. If in doubt—for example, following operation—this can be excluded by finding deep tendon reflexes, spinal withdrawal reflexes or by using a peripheral nerve stimulator.

In addition the cause of the patient's state must be known. This means both:

(1) Excluding metabolic disturbances by measurement of electrolytes (including Ca^{++}) and urea, blood glucose and acid base balance.
(2) Having a positive diagnosis of a disorder which can cause irreversible damage. When severe trauma or major intracerebral haemorrhage has occurred, tests for brain death may be delayed for not more than a few hours. However, when brain death is suspected after severe hypoxia, cardiac arrest or cere-

195

bral or fat embolism it is prudent to wait for 24 hours before making the first assessment.

The diagnosis should be made by two consultants or a consultant and senior registrar with expertise in the field working either together or separately. Needless to say, neither should belong to a transplant team if organ donation is anticipated. The tests should be carried out twice with the interval between being adequate for the re-assurance of all directly concerned.

The tests are as follows:

(1) Absent pupillary light reflex. The pupils may be either mid-point or dilated. The essential factor is that they are unreactive to light.
(2) Absent corneal reflex.
(3) Absent vestibulo-ocular reflex. If the eardrum is obscured by wax this must be removed. Slowly instill 20 ml of ice cold water into the external auditory canal. No eye movement (or other response) should occur. If the drum is obscured by local trauma this test can be omitted but the diagnosis of brain death still made if all the other conditions are fulfilled.
(4) Absent oculo-cephalic reflex (*see* p. 254).
(5) No gag or cough reflex on stimulation by catheter of the pharynx or trachea, respectively.
(6) No reaction in the area of distribution of the cranial nerves to a noxious stimulus. This may be conveniently applied by firm supraorbital or sternal pressure.
(7) No ventilatory response to hypercarbia. This is most conveniently assessed by ventilating the patient with pure oxygen for 10 minutes followed by 5% CO_2 in O_2 for 5 minutes. The patient is disconnected from the ventilator and observed for 10 minutes whilst delivering oxygen at 6 l/min by catheter into the endotracheal tube. This procedure will ensure that the Paco$_2$ will be at least 50 mmHg (6·65 kPa) whilst the patient is not exposed to additional hypoxia. If the patient has previous chronic respiratory failure and may normally exist on a hypoxic drive, expert advice should be sought on the test carried out with careful blood gas analysis.

A check list of these reflexes with recorded response is a useful aide memoire and entry for the notes.

Provided all these conditions are fulfilled:

(1) Other tests such as an EEG or arteriography are unnecessary and may only confuse distressed relatives.

(2) The decision to withdraw ventilation can be taken. The timing of this becomes increasingly irrelevant provided that all those concerned with the patient appreciate that he is already dead. In one institution it is the practice to issue a death certificate at this stage—whilst the patient is still being ventilated—in order to drive the point home. The timing must be balanced between unseemly haste and subsequent recrimination on the one hand and the needless prolongation of relatives uncertainty and suffering on the other.

SECTION VI REFERENCES

General

Adams RD, Victor M. *Principles of neurology*. New York: McGraw Hill, 1977.

Walton JN. *Brain's diseases of the nervous system 8th edition*. Oxford: Oxford Medical Publications, 1977

TIAs and stroke

1   Ackerman RH. Perspective of non-invasive diagnosis of carotid disease. *Neurology, Minneap* 1979; **29**: 615.

2   Beevers DG, Fairman MJ, Hamilton M, *et al.* Antihypertensive treatment and the course of established cerebral-vascular disease. *Lancet* 1973; **1**: 1407.

3   Fishman RA. Steroids in brain oedema. *N Engl J Med* 1982; **306**: 359.

4   Bohmfalk GL, Storey JL, Wissinger JP. Brown WE Jr. Bacterial intracranial aneurysm. *J Neurosurg* 1978; **48**: 369.

5   Canadian Co-operative Study Group. A randomised trial of aspirin and sulfinpyrazone in threatened stroke. *N Engl J Med* 1978; **299**: 53.

6   Collaborative group for the study of stroke in young women. Oral contraception and increased risk of cerebral ischaemia or thrombosis. *N Engl J Med* 1973; **288**: 871.

7   Fisher CM. Lacunes: small deep cerebral infarcts. *Neurology, Minneap* 1965; **15**: 774.

8   Genton E. Cerebral ischaemia: the role of thrombosis and antithrombotic therapy. *Stroke* 1977; **150**.

9   Leader. Mitral valve prolapse. *Br Med J* 1981; 1411.

10   Harrison MJG, Marshall J, Thomas DJ. Relevance of duration of transient ischaemic attacks in carotid territory. *Br Med J* 1978; **1**: 1578.

11   King T. Cerebral haemorrhage. *Br J Hosp Med* 1973; **10**: 250.

12   Leader. Treatment of acute cerebral infarction. *Br Med J* 1977; **1**: 1.

13   Leader. Aspirin and stroke prevention. *Lancet* 1978; **2**: 245.

14   Bartlett JR. Subarachnoid haemorrhage. *Br Med J* 1981; **2**: 1347.

15   Guarino JR. Auscultatory percussion of the head. *Br Med J* 1981; **1**: 1075.

16   Norris JW, Hachinski VC. Misdiagnosis of stroke. *Lancet* 1982; **1**: 328.
17   Leader. Ruptured intracranial aneurysm. *Lancet* 1979; **1**: 26.
18   McAllen PM, Marshall J. Cardiac dysrhythmia and transient cerebral ischaemic attacks. *Lancet* 1973; **1**: 1212.
19   Marshall J. Transient ischaemic attack. *Br J Hosp Med* 1973; **10**: 240.
20   Millikan CH. Treatment of transient ischaemic attacks. *Stroke* 1978; **9**: 299.
21   Mohr JP. Transient ischaemic attack and the prevention of strokes. *N Engl J Med* 1978; **299**: 93.
22   Naritomi H. Salzai F, Meyer JS, *et al.* Pathogenesis of transient ischaemic attacks within the vertebro-basilar arterial system. *Arch Neurology* 1979; **36**: 121.
23   Leader. Amaurosis fugax. *Lancet* 1982; **1**: 838.
24   Leader. Carotid stenosis. *Lancet* 1981; **1**: 535.
25   Ross Russell RW, Harrison MJG. The completed stroke. *Br J Hosp Med* 1973; **10**: 244.
26   Thomas DJ. Marshall J. Ross Russell RW. Effect of haematocrit on cerebral blood flow in man. *Lancet* 1977; **2**: 941.
27   Zervas MT. Subarachnoid haemorrhage. *N Engl J Med* 1978; **299**: 147.

Fits

28   Brown AS, Horton JM. Status epilepticus treated by intravenous infusions of thiopentone sodium. *Br Med J* 1967; **1**: 27.
29   Gastaut H. Courjon J, Poiré R, *et al.* Treatment of status epilepticus with a new benzodiazepine more active than diazepam. *Epilepsia* 1971; **12**: 197.
30   Greenblatt DJ, Shader RI, *et al.* Prazepam and lorazepan—two new benzodiazepines. *N Engl J Med* 1978; **299**: 1342.
31   Harvey PKP, Higenbottam TW, Loh L, *et al.* Chlormethiazole in treatment of status epilepticus. *Br Med J* 1975; **2**: 603.
32   Meldrum BS, Vigouroux RA, Brierley JB, *et al.* Systemic factors in epileptic brain damage: prolonged seizures in paralysed artificially ventilated baboons. *Arch Neurol* 1973; **27**: 82.
33   Swash M. Status epilepticus. *Br J Hosp Med* 1972; **8**: 269.

Acute ascending polyneuritis

34   Hewer RL, Hilton PJ, Smith AC. Acute polyneuritis requiring artificial ventilation. *Q J Med* 1968; **27**: 479.

35   Hughes RAC, Newsom-Davis JM, Perkin GD, Pierce JM. Controlled trial of prednisolone in acute polyneuropathy. *Lancet* 1978; **2**: 750.

Myasthenia gravis

36   Dau PC, Lindstrom JM, Lassel CK, Denys EH, Shev EE, Spitler LE. Therapy in myasthenia gravis. *N Engl J Med* 1977; **297**: 1134.
37   Drachman DB. Myasthenia gravis. *N Engl J Med* 1978; **298**: 136 and 186.
38   Leader. Plasmapheresis. *Br Med J* 1978; **1**: 1011.
39   Scadding GK, Harvard GWH. Pathogenesis and treatment of myasthenia gravis. *Br Med J* 1981; **2**: 1008.
40   Mann JD. The long-term administration of cortico-steroids and myasthenia gravis. *Neurology, Minneap* 1976; **26**: 729.

Tetanus

41   Weinstein L. Tetanus. *N Engl J Med* 1973; **289**: 1293.
42   Leader. Tetanus immune globulus: The intrathecal route. *Lancet* 1980; **2**: 464.

Brain death

43   Walker AE. Cerebral death. *Professional information library*.
44   Leader 1976.
45   Leader. Diagnosis of brain death. *Lancet* 1976; **2**: 1069.
46   Bolton CF, Brown JD, Cholod E, *et al*. EEG and 'brain life'. *Lancet* 1976; **1**: 535.
47   Black P McL. Brain death (two parts). *N Engl J Med* 1978; **299**: 338, 393.

SICKLE CELL ANAEMIA

Sickle cell anaemia[1]

(1) Sickle cell crisis does not occur in AS genotypes; it may be found in mixed haemoglobinopathies, such as SC disease, but more commonly it occurs in the homozygous sickle cell genotype. Distribution of the disease is throughout West Africa, the West Indies and North America, the Mediterranean littoral, and your patient will probably come from one of these areas.

(2) The basic problem is that deoxygenated haemoglobin tends to form gel precipitates in the red cell, causing them to sickle. Sickling is not necessarily irreversible, but the sickle cell is more sensitive to haemolysis, has a short life and, by increasing the viscosity of the blood, decreases flow in capillaries and small arterioles. The sickled cell also has a decreased oxygen carrying capacity.

(3) People suffering from sickle cell disease spend large portions of their life in a stable state, with mean haemoglobins of 9·0 g/100 ml. A crisis can be defined as a sharp turn or definite change in the course of the disease, with development of new signs and symptoms.

(4) Whatever the nature of the crisis, it is usually provoked by some stress, often an infection. This may be an urinary tract infection, diarrhoea and vomiting, pneumonia, or, in the tropics, malaria. Other provoking factors are exposure to cold, anaesthesia, operations and pregnancy.

(5) Four patterns of sickle cell crisis are described:

   (i) *Vaso-occlusive* (the commonest type). In this hyperviscosity causes sludging, stasis and infarction of the involved tissue. The symptoms are of a sudden onset of excruciating pain, often widespread, but most intense in one specific area. The commonest sites are the lumbo-sacral spine, chest, large joints and abdomen, where an intra-abdominal surgical crisis may be simulated. Because of the pain, your patient may be in agony. There will be widespread muscle and bone tenderness, an anaemia, a mild fever, and the white cell count is often raised to 20–60 000—even in the absence of infection. There may be a mild unconjugated hyperbilirubinaemia.

(ii)   *Haemolytic crisis*. Intravascular hypoxia causes a massive haemolysis. There will be profound anaemia (Hb 3–4 g/ 100 ml) and other features of haemolysis such as a reticulocytosis, low haptoglobin levels, and a raised indirect bilirubin.

(iii)   *Sequestration syndrome*. In this situation there is a sudden massive painful enlargement of the liver and spleen, probably on the basis of vaso-occlusive ischaemic damage to these organs. There is an acute fall in PCV, and Hb often falls to 2–3 g/100 ml. This type of crisis is restricted to children and pregnant women, and presents as cardiovascular collapse.

(iv)   *Aplastic or hypoplastic crisis*. There is abrupt cessation of function of the bone marrow, possibly again mediated through local ischaemia to the marrow. As in the haemolytic crisis there will be profound anaemia, but none of the other features of haemolysis.

Patients often have features of more than one of the above groups.

(6) There is, at present, no effective specific treatment which reverses sickling, although many remedies are being tried. The outcome of the sickle crisis largely depends on effective treatment of the underlying cause, which must be diligently sought.

TREATMENT

Take blood for FBP, a sickling screening test, blood gases, liver function tests, electrolytes and urea. Do blood cultures and where appropriate viral studies. Do an MSU and stool culture if there is diarrhoea. Do a chest x-ray and an ECG.

(1) The results of your history, examination and of the above tests should allow you to determine the underlying cause of the particular episode of crisis (*see* (4) above). This must be treated on its merits. Even if you don't find a specific cause, it is worth giving a broad spectrum antibiotic such as amoxycillin 250 mg eighthourly because of the frequent association of crisis and infection. You should also keep your patient warm.

(2) *Rehydration*. These patients are often fluid depleted, a factor which increases blood viscosity and thus hypoperfusion. Appropriate fluid, usually a mixture of 0·9% N saline and 5% dextrose should be infused under CVP control until the patient is

adequately perfused. The specific fluids you infuse will depend on the problem provoking the illness, and also on the results of your initial serum electrolytes.

(3) *Alkalis*. Acidosis is common in crisis, probably due to poor tissue perfusion. Acidosis also exacerbates sickling—thus it seems logical to reverse any acidosis present by giving $NaHCO_3$ as part of the infusion fluid, in amounts which you can calculate from the formula on page 246.

(4) *Oxygen*. Hypoxia also aggravates sickling and if the Pao_2 is below 80, it is reasonable to give 100% oxygen by face mask to correct this. Hyperbaric oxygen has been tried without success.

(5) *Pain relief*. The pain of crisis is severe and requires appropriate analgesics, opiates (pethidine 100 mg i.m., morphine 10 mg or diamorphine 5 mg i.m.) are often necessary. You should, of course, try simpler analgesics, such as aspirin and paracetamol first.

(6) *Correction of anaemia*. As mentioned above, 'sicklers' usually live with a Hb of around 9·0 g/100 ml. Unless there is profound anaemia (<6·0 g/100 ml) transfusion is unnecessary to raise the haemoglobin. However, partial exchange transfusions to replace some of the sickle cell haemoglobin with haemoglobin in the form of fresh heparinised blood has been suggested as a mode of treatment. There is no convincing evidence for its efficacy, but in desperate circumstances it is worth trying.

(7) *Specific anti-sickling drugs as therapeutic agents*. Advances in understanding of the theoretical basis of sickling have made possible several specific therapeutic approaches.[1, 2] So far none has been proven effective. However, as many of these treatments have been advocated, we feel that a brief survey of the mechanism and agents used is warranted, if only to warn against undue optimism.

Agents tried so far are:

(i) Compounds that prevent sickling by inhibiting intracellular gelation (gelation inhibitors) such as urea, dichloromethane gas, dimethyladipimidate and piracetam;

(ii) compounds which inhibit sickling independently of gelation—oral zinc cyanates; cysteamine therapy is said to be beneficial in the prevention of painful crisis.

We do not think that there is presently enough evidence to justify the use of any of these compounds.

SECTION VII REFERENCES

Sickle cell anaemia

1   Dean J, Schechter AN. Sickle cell anaemia. Molecular and cellular bases of therapeutic approaches. *N Engl J Med* 1978; **299**: 752 (part I); 804 (part II); 863 (part III).
2   Nalbandian RM, Henry RL, Murayama M, *et al.* Sickle cell disease. Two new strategies. *Lancet* 1978; **2**: 570.

THE OVERDOSE

The overdose[1,2,3,4]

DIAGNOSIS

(1) Usually rests on circumstantial or third party evidence and it is important therefore to interview relatives, ambulancemen, etc., and contact the patient's family doctor as soon as possible.
(2) Must be considered in any comatose patient.
(3) The effects may include:

    (i)   loss of consciousness to some degree, though not invariably;
    (ii) respiratory and cardiovascular depression;
    (iii) dehydration;
    (iv) hypothermia;
    (v) convulsions.

MANAGEMENT

This does not depend at the onset on the precise identification of the drugs involved. Measures in order of priority are:

(1) Clear and maintain an airway. Remove teeth, food, secretions, etc., and if necessary, insert an airway.
(2) Maintain respiration. The immediate need for assisted ventilation has to be assessed clinically but the efficiency of ventilation can only be gauged by measuring the blood gases. Retention of carbon dioxide ($Pa\text{co}_2$ of more than 45 mmHg) and hypoxia ($Pa\text{o}_2$ less than 70 mmHg) despite oxygen given by an MC face mask, are indications for artificial ventilation. It is unusual for a patient with a minute volume of greater than 4 l measured with a Wright spirometer, to require ventilation. But remember ventilatory function may fluctuate and can deteriorate suddenly.
(3) Maintenance of arterial pressure. If adequate tissue perfusion is not maintained:

    (i)   Put up a central venous pressure line and infuse plasma expanders and N saline in the usual way (*see* p. 277) until the CVP is in the upper range of normal. If this does not restore tissue perfusion, raise the systolic arterial pressure to above 85 mmHg by:

(ii) Dopamine, or failing this isoprenaline (*see* p. 13 for dosage of both these, and the section on the hypotensive patient for a more detailed account of the pathogenesis and management of shock in overdose patients).

(4) Treat arrhythmias (*see* p. 17).
(5) Correct hypothermia.
(6) General nursing care of the unconscious patient (*see* p. 260).
(7) Take blood and keep urine for drug analysis.
(8) When all this has been instituted consider measures designed to remove the substance from the body.

(i) A stomach washout seems a logical measure in any patient who has taken a potentially toxic dose of poison. However, it is unproductive if performed more than 4 hours after the tablets have been taken—except in poisoning from salicylates, tricyclic antidepressants and antispasmodic agents, when it is worth doing up to 12 hours. If the patient is unconscious, consent for this must be obtained, and if he or she persists in witholding consent, so be it. It is dangerous to perform a stomach washout on the unconscious patient without having an endotracheal tube in place. Put the patient in the head down position and pass a well lubricated 30–40 French gauge orogastric tube into the stomach (it is virtually impossible to pass a large bore tube direct into the trachea). Aspirate the stomach contents and introduce 250 ml of luke-warm water. Leave 2–3 minutes and then re-aspirate. Repeat this procedure until 2 l have been used. If laryngeal spasm occurs during gastric lavage, some inhalation of stomach contents has probably occurred. In this case aspirate the remainder of the stomach contents and withdraw the tube. If serious inhalation of stomach contents occurs, you should give hydrocortisone 200 mg i.v., oxygen as necessary, broad spectrum antibiotics, including one effective against anaerobes (*see* p. 249) institute suction and physiotherapy, and treat wheezing as for asthma (*see* p. 70).

Gastric lavage should not be undertaken in any patient who has taken petroleum distillates (for fear of inhalation of these occurring). In patients who have taken corrosives, lavage should only be used if there is a serious danger of systemic effects developing from these corrosives, as in the case of formic acid and Paraquat.

Some authorities now favour inducing emesis as an alternative to gastric lavage. Syrup of ipecacuanha, in a dose of 30 ml for adults, is an effective way of so doing.

Induction of vomiting is contra-indicated in poisoning due to corrosives, petroleum distillates, anti-emetics(!) and in anyone whose conscious level is impaired.

As a general rule the above measures are all that is required in management of overdoses. However, there are a few specific occasions when something further can be done, and these are discussed below; and in ensuing directions (q.v.).

(ii) A forced diuresis may be worth doing in the following:

    (a) long acting barbiturates (*see* below);
    (b) primidone;
    (c) salicylates (*see* below);
    (d) amphetamines—the excretion of which is promoted by an acid diuresis;
    (e) lithium;
    (f) methyl alcohol—although haemodialysis, with appropriate correction of the extreme acidosis is more effective in this condition (*see* (vi) below);
    (g) Quinine and phencyclidine ('angel dust')—whose excretion is promoted by an acid diuresis.

(iii) Orally administered absorbents may have an occasional role. Activated charcoal (medicoal) in a dose of 5–10 g should be given in tricyclic antidepressant poisoning, and in ingestion of some other less common agents such as theophylline, phenothiazines and antihistamines.[6]

(iv) Forced diuresis has been advocated for both phenytoin and ethyl alcohol, but results are not encouraging, and we do not use it for these substances.

(v) Haemoperfusion over activated charcoal or resin is an efficient and safe method of removing at least all types of barbiturates, glutethimide and salicylates from the body. Where available, it is the treatment of choice for severely intoxicated patients who fail to respond to supportive measures.[5]

(vi) Haemodialysis—only removes substances which are water soluble and which the kidney can likewise excrete. Effective forced diuresis is as efficient as haemodialysis, which should therefore only be used if there is renal failure, if charcoal haemoperfusion is not available, or in methyl alcohol poisoning.

(9) *Naloxone*. This is a specific antidote for morphine and morphine-like compounds. It acts immediately (within five minutes) and its effect will be dramatic if your patient has taken an opiate or opiate derivative (including codeine, dextropropoxyphene and pentazocine). It will not do any harm if your patient turns out to have taken some other substance. Thus if there is uncertainty as to which drug has been taken in any overdose with poor perfusion and poor respiration, naloxone (0·4 mg–1·2 mg i.v. over 3 minutes) should be used both as a diagnostic and therapeutic agent.

(10) Information as to the constituents of compounds and advice as to the management of their ingestion may be had from the following Poisons Information Centres:

Belfast:	The Royal Victoria Hospital	
		Tel: 0232 40503
Cardiff:	Royal Infirmary	0222 492233
Dublin:	Jervis Street Hospital	0001 745588
Edinburgh:	Royal Infirmary	031 229 2477
London:	Guy's Hospital	01 407 7600

(11) All these measures, complicated as they are, only constitute first aid and are relatively simple compared to the patient's problems on regaining consciousness.

Salicylates

Twenty-five grams is the fatal dose in adults but death can occur from lesser doses. One aspirin tablet (BP) contains 300 mg.

DIAGNOSIS

The patient is confused, restless, flushed, sweating, hyperventilating and complains of tinnitus. Coma is unusual unless a really massive and frequently fatal overdose has been absorbed. The following metabolic changes may be present.

(1) A hypokalaemic alkalosis caused by vomiting.
(2) A respiratory alkalosis (low P_{aCO_2} high bicarbonate) caused by hyperventilation.
(3) A metabolic acidosis possibly caused by absorption of acid, dehydration and poor peripheral glucose metabolism.
(4) Dehydration, caused by hyperventilation, sweating, vomiting and reduced fluid intake.
(5) Hypo or hyperglycaemia.
(6) A bleeding tendency—usually due to hypoprothrombinaemia, plus decreased platelet adhesiveness.
(7) Pulmonary oedema—a hypersensitivity phenomenon which thus gives rise to the shock lung syndrome (see p. 83).

In children either the acidosis or the alkalosis may predominate;adults are nearly always alkalotic when first seen. The clinical state is due to combination of the direct effect of salicylates, dehydration and the acid/base status.

MANAGEMENT

Salicylate poisoning is one of the few overdose conditions where early measurement of blood levels is very useful. Some patients with high blood levels show little clinical evidence of it and yet are in great danger. Symptoms occur at about 1·9 mmol (30 mg/100 ml). The intoxication is reckoned as severe if the level is more than 3·1 mmol (50 mg/100 ml) and a forced alkaline diuresis is then indicated.[8]

Charcoal haemoperfusion or, failing that, haemodialysis may be indicated if the level is more than 6·2 mmol (100 mg%) (or if more than 4·3 mmol (70 mg%) and the level is rising rapidly), or if the patient is in coma, or if there is impairment of renal function.

One value does not necessarily act as a guide to management. Far more useful are levels taken at regular intervals, e.g. every 6 hours. Finally, do not rely on the blood levels alone. The most important guide to the severity of the poisoning is the patient's condition. If it is bad and deteriorating then energetic measures should be instituted whatever the level.

(1) Take blood for serum salicylate, haemoglobin and PCV, electrolytes and urea, arterial pH and Paco$_2$. Of these results the arterial pH is needed first. Urine should be tested for the presence of salicylates. They act as a reducing substance in Benedict's test even after the urine has been boiled (*see* p. 133). A simple 'side ward' test has been described for the estimate of plasma salicylate levels.[7]

(2) Give vitamin K, 15 mg i.m.

(3) A forced alkaline diuresis should be started if:

   (i)   the clinical condition is poor, i.e. the signs above are marked;
   (ii) the salicylate level is more than 1·9 mmol (30 mg%) in children and more than 3·1 mmol (50 mg%) in adults;
   (iii) there is a history of ingestion of more than 50 tablets.

(4) Alkalinisation is unnecessary if the urine pH is already more than 8 and is dangerous if the arterial pH is more than 7·5. In either of these situations merely start a forced diuresis (*see* below). If the urine pH remains acid in the face of an apparent arterial alkalosis there is usually intracellular potassium depletion. Until this is corrected by potassium supplements, it is difficult to achieve production of an alkaline urine.

(5) If the indications for forced diuresis are absent simply observe the patient closely and encourage oral fluids.

(6) If pulmonary oedema occurs manage as for shock lung (*see* p. 83).

Forced diuresis—alkaline and acid

(1) Catheterise the bladder and keep the urine.

(2) Set up a central venous pressure line (*see* p. 275) and when it reads within the normal range (you may have to give i.v. saline and dextrose to achieve this) assess the rate of urine flow.

(3) If the rate of urine flow is above 4 ml/min with the patient adequately perfused, you may start the forced diuresis; if the urine flow is less than this, give frusemide 20 mg i.v. If the frusemide produces a urine flow of greater than 4 ml/min it is safe to start the diuresis. If after the frusemide the urine flow is less than 4 ml/min, it is likely that renal insufficiency is present, and the diuresis should not be undertaken. If you consider it safe to carry out the diuresis, proceed in rotation, with the following infusions:

> 1·26% NaHCO$_3$—500 ml (90 mmol NaHCO$_3$)
> 5% dextrose—500 ml
> 5% dextrose—500 ml
> 0·9% N saline—500 ml

Do not give the bicarbonate until the arterial pH is known. Give 1 litre of this regime each hour for 6 hours, and 500 ml/hour thereafter. Provided the patient was adequately perfused prior to starting the diuresis (which, as pointed out in (2) above, may require an initial infusion of up to 5 litres of N saline and 5% dextrose), urine output should approximate fluid input. If this is not the case, give i.v. frusemide, 20 mg as needed to keep the urine output up. If, after frusemide, the urinary output does not go up, or if the patient develops fluid overload, it is probable that a degree of renal impairment is present (but check that the urinary catheter isn't blocked!). The diuresis should therefore be stopped, and charcoal haemoperfusion or haemodialysis considered. For a forced diuresis, rather than a forced alkaline diuresis, merely substitute 0·45 N saline for the 1·2% NaHCO$_3$ and proceed as above. To induce an acid diuresis, you should give 10 g of arginine or lysine hydrochloride i.v. over 30 minutes, and then give oral ammonium chloride 4 g two-hourly as necessary to keep the urine pH between 5·5 and 6·5.

(4) Give K$^+$ 26 mmol with each litre of fluid to start with.

215

(5) Measure and chart:

    (i)   the total fluid input and the fluid output with a cumulative total every hour;

    (ii)   the central venous pressure every 30 minutes;

    (iii)   the urine pH hourly (if possible on a pH meter, which is more accurate than the universal indicator strip)— Remember the achievement of an alkaline urine is as important as the high urine output, and you must act on the regular pH readings;

    (iv)   the urinary and blood electrolytes and urea, and the arterial pH and Paco$_2$ every 4 hours;

    (v)   the serum salicylate every 6 hours whilst the patient's condition is critical.

(6) The intensive monitoring is necessary because salicylate intoxication is one of the most complex metabolic states you will have to treat, and because a necessary forced diuresis, if not carefully watched, can be extremely dangerous. It follows therefore that the patient should be transferred to a centre where this is possible.

These measurements will allow for the following adjustments:

    (i)   Fluid (*see* above).

    (ii)   As soon as the urine pH is above 8, substitute 0·5 N saline for the bicarbonate.

    (iii)   If hyponatraemia is developing, substitute N saline for one of the bottles of 5% dextrose.

    (iv)   Replace the measured potassium loss in the urine over 4 hours at the end of which time re-measure and repeat the process.

(7) Continue this regime, repeating the serum salicylate level, urinary and serum electrolytes and urea every 6 hours. Similarly, the arterial pH and Paco should be measured six-hourly until the serum salicylate level is less than 3·1 mmol/1 (50 mg%).

(8) If the diuresis continues for more than 6 hours give 10 ml of 10% calcium gluconate six-hourly. This will protect your patient against hypocalcaemic tetany, an occasional complication of prolonged alkaline diuresis.

Barbiturates

DIAGNOSIS

Is from other forms of overdose and other causes of coma (*see* p. 253). A simple method for assessing blood barbiturate levels should be available to you through your biochemical laboratory.

MANAGEMENT

(1) Very few patients with barbiturate poisoning need more than supportive management. The mortality in those seriously affected is often due to irreversible changes, e.g. cerebral infarction, sustained before starting treatment. It can also be due to over-energetic treatment.

(2) Charcoal haemoperfusion is probably the treatment of choice for all severe barbiturate overdoses (*see* p. 211).

(3) If charcoal haemoperfusion is not available, forced alkaline diuresis (*see* p. 215) is only indicated for substantial overdoses of phenobarbitone and barbitone. For all the other barbiturates, it is of no avail.

(4) The decision to undertake charcoal haemoperfusion or a forced diuresis is primarily a clinical one. The indications are:

    (i)   A history of considerable ingestion coupled with a rapidly deteriorating patient.

    (ii)   A patient who is sufficiently unconscious that there is no response to pain (as produced by rubbing the knuckles over the patient's sternum). The pupillary and tendon reflexes are very variable and frequently lead one to suppose that the patient is more severely poisoned than he actually is. Inadequacy of the patient's spontaneous respiratory efforts and hypotension occurring in the absence of hypovolaemia are also sinister signs.

    (iii) If the patient's clinical state deteriorates markedly in the face of rising or static blood barbiturate levels (*see* below).

Provided that reliable laboratory techniques are available, the blood barbiturate level must be carried out as a high level may act as a warning of the seriousness of the situation, viz. over 0·21 mmol (5 mg/100 ml) for short and medium acting barbiturates and 0·43 mmol (10 mg/100 ml) for phenobarbitone.

(5) There is no place for the use of bemegride, at one time thought to be a specific barbiturate antagonist. In fact, its use has been associated with increased mortality.

Digoxin

For this widely prescribed drug acute overdosage is rare, but toxicity may readily arise from its therapeutic use. The maximal therapeutic dose is about 60% of the minimal toxic dose and toxicity is especially likely to occur:

    (i)   if diuretics are given without potassium supplements;
    (ii) after a bout of diarrhoea or vomiting (both of which may cause K^+ depletion);
    (iii) if the patient is old and/or small;
    (iv) if the patient has renal or hepatic failure;
    (v) if other drugs, e.g. morphine, are being taken.

DIAGNOSIS

The patient may complain of vomiting and diarrhoea (which may exacerbate a pre-existing hypokalaemia) visual disturbances (blurring, flashes of light and xanthopsia), and the effects of almost any cardiac arrhythmia, the commonest being atrioventricular block, supraventricular tachycardia, ventricular ectopics and ventricular tachycardia.

Clinically, digoxin toxicity may be difficult to distinguish from the underlying heart disorder for which it was prescribed (*see* p. 18). Blood levels may be helpful, provided the blood sample is taken 6 hours after the last oral dose, the normal therapeutic range being 1·0–2·0 mg/ml ($<2 \mu g/l$).

MANAGEMENT

(1) If the patient is nauseated and is having occasional ventricular ectopics it is usually sufficient to discontinue the drug for a day or two. The effect of digoxin can be partially reversed by potassium, and 20–40 mmol of KCl per day orally should be given.

(2) If the situation is more urgent (e.g. the patient has persistent vomiting, is in heart failure, heart block or has an arrhythmia

compromising output) the following two measures should be instituted.

(i)   i.v. K^+ should be given .40 mmol K^+ in 5% dextrose should be infused over 1 hour, with continuous ECG monitoring. The drip should be stopped immediately if sinus rhythm returns or if peaking of T waves (evidence of hyperkalaemia) occurs. Up to 120 mmol K^+ may have to be given. If the initial serum K^+ was normal, it is wise to infuse the K^+ in a 500 ml solution of 33% dextrose with 30 units of soluble insulin added.

(ii) Magnesium also counteracts the toxic effects of digoxin on the myocardium. Therefore, as well as giving K^+, give 2 ml of 50% $MgSO_4$ diluted to 50 cc over the course of 1 hour, and repeat as necessary.

(3) If the above therapy is unsuccessful further treatment will be required. Propranolol 1–2 mg i.v. slowly is said to be the drug of choice for digoxin-induced ectopics and tachycardias.

Atropine 0·6 mg i.v. may counteract digoxin-induced bradycardias. Transvenous pacing may be required for persistent heart block, or a widening PR interval despite K^+ therapy.

(4) In patients with digoxin-induced arrhythmias D.C. reversion may provoke either heart block, or, rarely, resistant ventricular tachycardia. So cardioversion should not be used lightly in such patients. However, in the face of a life-threatening arrhythmia, D.C. reversion (see p. 19) should be undertaken. Transvenous pacing will be required if heart block occurs, and so should be readily available.

(5) Digoxin undergoes an enterohepatic circulation, and cholestyramine can bind it in the gut. This provides a possible, but as yet untested, way of getting rid of digoxin.

(6) Incomplete (Fab fragment) anti-digoxin antibodies have the advantage of nullifying the effect of digoxin without being immunogenic.[9] Not yet generally available, they may ultimately provide the most satisfactory answer to this problem.

Iron[10]

Some iron tablets look like certain well-known sweets, and sometimes small children unwittingly take handfuls of them. A dose of 3 g as elemental iron may be fatal (a 200 mg tablet of ferrous sulphate contains 60 mg and a 300 mg tablet of ferrous gluconate contains 36 mg of elemental iron). The features of iron poisoning are:

(1) Acute haemorrhagic gastroenteritis up to 3 hours after ingestion and then often after a spurious interval of apparent spontaneous recovery.
(2) Acute encephalopathy (up to 24 hours).
(3) Occasionally acute hepatic necrosis (up to 3 days).
(4) Following recovery from these reactions there may be subsequent cicatricial strictures of the gut.

MANAGEMENT

If treatment is started as soon as possible the complications of (2) and (3) above may be avoided.

(1) Give desferrioxamine 2 g i.m.
(2) Wash out the stomach and leave behind desferrioxamine 5–10 g in 50 ml of fluid.
(3) Take blood for haemoglobin and PCV electrolytes and urea and serum iron.
(4) If a history of ingestion of considerable quantities is obtained or vomiting or bloody diarrhoea occurs, or serum iron is above 90 μmol/1 (500 μg%) give desferrioxamine 15 mg/kg/hour i.v. to a maximum of 80mg/kg/24 hour. This, if necessary, may be infused added to blood.
(5) Continue giving desferrioxamine 2 g i.m. 12-hourly until the serum iron is less than 90 μmol/l (500 μg%) and the clinical state is satisfactory. This will have to be continued for 24 hours as iron which is initially taken up by the reticulo-endothelial system is released 12 hours later.
(6) Blood may need to be given if haemorrhage has been severe. 0·9% N saline, 5% dextrose and potassium supplements may need to be given if diarrhoea has been severe.

Tricyclic and tetracyclic antidepressants

Today, drugs of this group are amongst the most commonly taken in overdose. Clinical features include depression of consciousness, which is seldom severe, dilated and sometimes unequal pupils responding poorly to light, increased muscle tone which may be accompanied by tremor or frank convulsions, pronounced tendon reflexes and urinary retention. Additionally, cardiac dysrhythmias are an important feature of overdose in this group of drugs.

MANAGEMENT

(1) Is essentially supportive care as outlined on page 209, as there is no known way of accelerating elimination of these drugs.
(2) Prompt and adequate correction of any acidosis by giving appropriate doses of bicarbonate intravenously.[12]
(3) Monitor ECG—only if cardiac irregularities persist in spite of institution of measures outlined in (1) and (2) should conventional anti-arrhythmics be employed. Neostigmine 0·25 mg i.v. at 5-minute intervals to a maximum of 2·5 mg has been advocated for supraventricular tachycardia in this situation, but its advantage over other anti-arrhythmics is doubtful.
(4) It is likely that 10 g of effervescent charcoal taken orally (or by a n.g. tube if the patient is unconscious) will absorb any residual drug in the GI tract, and thus minimise any absorbtion which might take place after you first see the patient.[11]
(5) Convulsions should be controlled without delay by conventional means (*see* p. 182).

Paracetamol

Overdoses (e.g. 15 g or more) of this drug which only give rise to nausea as an initial symptom, may later cause acute hepatic necrosis.[14] Approximate blood levels, after which hepatic necrosis is likely, are given in Fig. 22. If these blood levels are exceeded, treatment with specific antidotes should be considered.[15]

(1) Most conveniently, methionine orally with 2·5 g as the initial dose, followed by three more doses, each of 2·5 g at four-hourly intervals. If your patient is vomiting, or oral methionine is not available, use N-acetylcysteine (*see* below).

(2) Alternative, N-acetylcysteine by the intravenous route at a dose initially of 150 mg per kg body weight in 200 ml 5% dextrose over 15 minutes, followed over the next 4 hours by a second dose of 50 mg per kg body weight in 0·5 litre of 5% dextrose and finally over 16 hours, a dose of 100 mg per kg body weight in 1 litre of 5% dextrose.[16]

(3) Thirdly, if either of the above are not available intravenous cysteamine may be administered, first a dose of 2 g over 10 minutes, and then 400 mg in 500 ml dextrose four-hourly for 12 hours.

If more than 10 hours have elapsed since ingestion the use of a specific antidote is contra-indicated, for it is unlikely to be effective, and indeed, may be harmful. In these circumstances, haemoperfusion over activated charcoal should be considered.

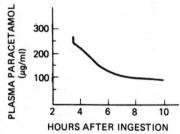

Fig. 22. Plasma paracetamol concentrations after overdosage. Treatment is indicated in patients with concentrations exceeding those shown in the graph. By permission of Prescott L. F. *et al.*, and the editors of *The Lancet*.

Distalgesic[17]

This analgesic is being prescribed, and thus also being taken in overdose, with increasing frequency. All this despite the fact that there is little evidence that it is in any way superior to other simple analgesics. Each table contains 32·5 mg dextropropoxyphene and 325 mg paracetamol.

MANAGEMENT

(1) Dextropropoxyphene is closely related to methadone, and thus any cardio-respiratory depressant effects are reversible with naxolone (*see* p. 261).
(2) The paracetamol level should be measured, and appropriate therapy started (*see* p. 223).

SECTION VIII REFERENCES

General

1 Vale JA, Meredith TJ. *Poisoning diagnosis and treatment.* Update Books, 1981.
2 Goulding R. Drug overdosage. *Br J Hosp Med* 1972; **8**: 293.
3 Mathew H. Acute poisoning. Some myths and misconceptions. *Br Med J* 1971; **1**: 519.
4 Stengel E. Suicide. *Hospital Medicine* 1968; **2**: 1058.
5 Vale JA, Rees AJ, Widdop B, Goulding R. The use of charcoal haemoperfusion in the management of severely poisoned patients. *Br Med J* 1975; **1**: 5.
6 Leader. Medicoal (effervescent activated charcoal) in the treatment of acute poisoning. *Drug Ther Bull* 1979; **17**: 2.

Specific agents

Salicylates

7 Brown SS, Smith AC, Salicylate estimation in the side room. *Br Med J* 1968; **4**: 327.
8 Lawson AAH. Forced diuresis in the treatment of acute salicylate poisoning in adults. *Q J Med* 1969; **138**: 31.

Digoxin

9 Smith TW, Haber E, Yeatman L, *et al.* Reversal of advanced digoxin intoxication with Fab fragments of digoxin-specific anti-bodies. *N Engl J Med* 1976; **294**: 797.

Iron

10 Lavender S. Iron intoxication in an adult. *Br Med J* 1970; **2**: 406.

Tricyclic antidepressants

11 Crome P, Dawling S, Braithwaite RA, Masters J, Walkey R. Effect of activated charcoal on absorption of nortriptylene. *Lancet* 1977; **2**: 1203.
12 Leader. Sodium bicarbonate and tricyclic antidepressant poisoning. *Lancet* 1976; **2**: 838.

225

Paracetamol

13 Crome P, Vale JA, Volans GN, *et al*. Oral methionine in the treatment of severe paracetamol (acetaminophen) overdose. *Lancet* 1976; **2**: 829.

14 Leader. Paracetamol hepatotoxicity. *Lancet* 1975; **2**: 1189.

15 Prescott LF, Roscoe P, Wright N, *et al*. Plasma paracetamol half life and hepatic necrosis in patients with paracetamol overdosage. *Lancet* 1971; **1**: 519.

16 Prescott LF, Illingworth RN, Critchley JAJH, Stewart MJ, Adam RD, Proudfoot AT. Intravenous N-acetylcysteine: the treatment of choice for paracetamol poisoning. *Br Med J* 1979; **2**: 1097.

Dextropropoxyphene

17 Leader. Treatment of dextropropoxyphene poisoning. *Lancet* 1977; **2**: 542.

HYPOTHERMIA

Hypothermia[2,3,4]

Hypothermia has been defined as a central (usually rectal) temperature of less than 35°C (95°F).

DIAGNOSIS

(1) Hypothermia can only be diagnosed using a low reading rectal thermometer. A recording of 33°C should arouse suspicion and the true temperature may be lower as this is the lowest reading on an ordinary thermometer.

(2) Hypothermia may be the sole cause of coma in anyone exposed to a low temperature.

(3) Alternatively it may complicate coma from other causes— especially hypoglycaemia, strokes, alcohol and chlorpromazine overdosage. It may either precipitate or be caused by myxoedema (*see* p. 153) and hypopituitary coma (*see* p. 147).

(4) Below about 31°C (88°F) shivering gives way to muscular rigidity accompanied by a slow pulse and respiration and hypotension. Acidosis, caused by hypoventilation and excessive lactic acid production, may be present. The ECG shows J (junctional) waves[1] (Fig. 23). Ventricular fibrillation can occur at any temperature below 30°C (86°F).

MANAGEMENT

Take blood for full blood count, electrolytes and urea, serum amylase, blood glucose, blood gases and thyroid function. Measure the rectal temperature half-hourly. Further measures are:

(i) The general care of the unconscious patient (*see* p. 260).
(ii) Treatment of the hypothermia and its complications.

(1) If hypothermia occurs in a young patient as an acute episode as, for example, immersion in cold water, put the patient in a bath at 56°C (113°F) and then into a bed with warm blankets.

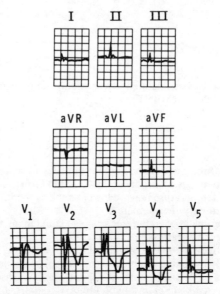

Fig. 23. The ECG in hypothermia. By permission of the authors, Drs D. Emslie-Smith, G. E. Sladden and G. Stirling, and the publishers of the *British Heart Journal*.

(2) In other circumstances controversy over the rate of re-warming still exists. Traditionally, slow warming (0·8°C per hour) has been advocated. This is achieved by nursing the patient covered with blankets in a room at 26–29°C. However, the morbidity from hypothermia is directly related to the time spent hypothermic. Therefore, more rapid warming at a rate of about 1·5°C per hour may be advisable though careful nursing, preferably in an ITU is essential. In any case look out for these factors which can complicate hypothermia (*see* (iii) below).

(3) Coma may be complicated by:

    (i)   Hypotension. This may be caused by:

        (a) Steroid insufficiency. Take blood for a cortisol level and then give 200 mg of hydrocortisone i.v. followed by 50 mg i.v. four-hourly if there is an initial response.

(b) Relative circulatory insufficiency produced by peripheral vasodilation as re-warming proceeds. If necessary put up a CVP line and infuse plasma in the usual way (*see* p. 277) until the CVP is normal.

Avoid using catecholamines in this condition if possible—they are especially likely to cause ventricular arrhythmias.

(ii) Hypoventilation. This may need treatment (indicated as always by measurement of the blood gases). Hypothermia may lead to dependence on hypoxic drive (as in some patients with chronic respiratory failure) and artificial ventilation may be necessary.

(iii) Acidosis which may be severe. Calculate the base deficit (*see* p. 246) and restore with the appropriate amount of sodium bicarbonate in the usual way.

(iv) Ventricular fibrillation. As the oxygen demand of tissues is reduced in this condition, it may be worthwhile continuing cardiac massage for longer than usual. If ordinary methods of d.c. reversion do not cause a return to sinus rhythm it has been suggested that a thoracotomy should be performed and the pericardium irrigated with warm saline—internal defibrillation then being attempted.

(v) Pulmonary oedema is an occasional complication of rewarming, due to leaky capillaries, and thus really a form of 'shock lung' (*see* p. 83). Intermittent positive pressure ventilation may be necessary.

(vi) Infection. A broad spectrum antibiotic should be given i.v. as pneumonia usually develops.

(vii) Acute pancreatitis—the incidence of which is overestimated.

SECTION IX REFERENCES

Hypothermia

1   Emslie-Smith D, Sladden GE, Stirling GR. The significance of changes in the ECG in hypothermia. *Br J Hosp Med* 1959; **21**: 343.
2   Exton-Smith AM. Accidental hypothermia. *Br Med J* 1973; **4**: 727.
3   Hervey GR. Physiological changes occurring in hypothermia. *Proc R Soc Med* 1973; **66**: 1053.
4   Leader. Treating accidental hypothermia. *Br Med J* 1978; **2**: 1383.

GENERAL CLINICAL PROBLEMS

The uncontrolled and potentially hostile patient

Sudden onset of mental deterioration must be considered an emergency, and constitutes one of the severest tests of clinical skills.

DIAGNOSIS

The following conditions must always be borne in mind:

(1) Cerebral hypoxia (poor perfusion, or poor oxygenation).
(2) Infection—any, but particularly meningitis, encephalitis, pneumonia (especially pneumococcal) and septicaemia.
(3) Any pain or discomfort (commonly urinary retention) in a patient already seriously ill.
(4) Drugs—the following most frequently: barbiturates (especially in the elderly), amphetamines, monoamine oxidase inhibitors, atropine, corticosteroids, anti-Parkinson drugs, and ephedrine. Almost every drug has been implicated at some time.
(5) An intracranial space-occupying lesion, e.g. tumour, abscess or haematoma—either extra-dural, sub-dural or intracerebral.
(6) Hypoglycaemia or more rarely, hyperglycaemia.
(7) Alcohol, either its excess or its sudden withdrawal (*see* p. 238).
(8) Complex partial seizures, such as may occur in temporal lobe epilepsy.
(9) Myxoedema (*see* p. 153).
(10) Thyrotoxicosis (*see* p. 155).
(11) SLE.
(12) Deficiency of thiamine, (Wernickes encephalopathy—external ophthalmoplegia, ataxia and confusion), nicotinamide and vitamin B_{12}.
(13) Hypo or hypernatraemia.
(14) Hypokalaemia.
(15) Hepatic pre-coma (*see* p. 110).
(16) Hypo or hypercalcaemia (*see* pp. 160, 158).
(17) Acute porphyria.

Two or more of these may occur together. Any may be exacerbated by anaemia, hypotension or pre-existing chronic dementia.

MANAGEMENT

(1) Involves consideration of the above causes. As a routine you must ask for:

   (i)   haemoglobin and PCV;
   (ii)   electrolytes and urea;
   (iii) blood sugar;
   (iv)   blood calcium;
   (v)   blood gases;
   (vi)   skull x-ray;
   and take a careful drug history.

(2) Confusion is always worse at night. Disorientation may be helped by an easily visible clock, a familiar nurse and a light.

(3) (i)   Never attempt to sedate an uncontrolled patient without due consideration of the cause, it may make the situation worse and it may be fatal. If sedation is vital or is deemed unharmful give chlorpromazine (50–100 mg i.m.) initially or phenobarbitone 100 mg i.m. or diazepam 10 mg i.m.

   (ii)   If the above are ineffective give either

       (a) chlormethiazole (*see* p. 239);

           or

       (b) a cocktail of haloperidol 20 mg;
           kemadrin 20 mg;
           promethazine (sparine) 100 mg;
           all intra-muscularly—and drawn up in the same syringe.

This rarely fails to bring peace to the patient and his attendants. Never give paraldehyde to a confused but conscious patient as the pain provides considerable force and direction for the structure of his delusions. It goes without saying that your verbal or pharmacological attempts to calm the patient must not be attended by any hint of aggression. It not only betrays lack of insight on your part, it may also be the only face of your relationship to be grasped by the patient— and is therefore disastrous.

Acute psychoses

DIAGNOSIS

The clinical picture may be very similar to some of the conditions described on p. 235 and if in doubt you must do at least (1) (i)–(vi) on p. 236. In addition, sudden medical or surgical illness may provoke an acute psychosis in a sufficiently susceptible patient. A history of previous mental illness may therefore be present. A helpful point of distinction between an acute psychosis and a toxic confusional state is that in the former the sensorium is clear, although the content of thought is disordered.

Consider:

(1) Puerperal psychosis.
(2) Acute schizophrenia. Usually presents a characteristic mixture of disorders of thinking and feelings, with hallucinations and disorders of conduct. This closely resembles the picture of amphetamine psychosis.
(3) Acute depression. Delusions and hallucinations are usually of a self-deprecatory nature. Hypochondriasis, suicidal ruminations and a tendency to depersonalisation may be evident.
(4) Acute mania. Elation combines characteristically with easily provoked irritability. The patient talks rapidly, jumping from one subject to another.
(5) Acute hysterical episodes. Overtones of acting and self-dramatisation may be apparent. Even when at his most violent the patient rarely injures himself.

MANAGEMENT

Involves:

(1) Achieving, if at all possible, some kind of contact with the patient, if only to establish yourself as a harmless and possibly helpful comrade.
(2) Consideration of the general principles as outlined in sections (2) and (3) on p. 236.
(3) Initiating the treatment of specific psychiatric syndromes.
(4) Psychiatric consultation which should be sought as soon as possible.

Toxic confusional state due to acute alcohol withdrawal[1]—delirium tremens

Acute withdrawal from alcohol causes a characteristic toxic confusional state, which, if uncontrolled, may be fatal.

DIAGNOSIS

(1) DTs usually occur in a patient who has been withdrawn suddenly from alcohol after a binge lasting at least two weeks, and often considerably longer.

(2) The characteristic symptoms are tremulousness, apprehension, disorientation in time and place and visual, tactile and auditory hallucinations. In addition, insomnia, nausea and vomiting and motor inco-ordination may be present.

(3) These symptoms usually begin within hours of withdrawal, and are maximal from about 24–48 hours. Their occurrence should be anticipated in persons known to be heavy drinkers.

(4) Excessive intake of alcohol may also give rise to cirrhosis, cardiomyopathy and various neurological syndromes such as peripheral neuropathy due to vitamin deficiency, chronic cerebellar disease and Wernicke's encephalopathy. Thus, DTs may be superimposed on an already debilitated patient.

MANAGEMENT

(1) Non-specific:

    (i)   It is very important to establish contact with the patient who is frightened, disorientated and frequently aggressive. A sympathetic, understanding approach is mandatory and usually successful.

    (ii)   Thiamine 50 mg i.v. and 50 mg i.m. should always be given before starting a dextrose infusion thereby avoiding the possibility of precipitating Wernicke's encephalopathy in a susceptible patient.

(2) Specific:

(i) The aim of treatment is the induction of light sleep sufficient to control symptoms, whilst leaving vital functions unimpaired. Drugs to achieve this end are best given orally, but may have to be given i.v.

(ii) Chlormethiazole (Heminevrin) is the drug of choice. The dose required to achieve (i) above ranges between 4·0 and 10·0 g/day. It requires being reviewed daily, the highest dose generally being needed 24–48 hours after alcohol withdrawal. Patients generally do not need this drug after the seventh day. If oral administration is impossible, i.v. chlormethiazole may be given. Give a loading dose of 30–50 ml of a 0·8% solution over 3–5 minutes to induce sleep, and continue an infusion of this concentration at 0·5–1·0 ml/min, adjusting the rate to keep the patient just sleeping lightly. Usually 500–1000 ml are needed in the first 6–12 hours. Chlormethiazole is a very safe drug. Side-effects, which are dose-related, are respiratory depression, hypotension and supra-ventricular tachycardia.

(iii) Chlordiazepoxide, either orally or i.v. in sufficient dosage necessary to induce light sleep may be used as an alternative to chlormethiazole. Start with 40 mg four-hourly and increase to 100 mg two-hourly if necessary.

(iv) Although the tremulousness, fever, tachycardia, and hallucinations subside over three to four days, there may be an interval over 1–2 weeks before full return to the patient's previous mental state. This interval is characterised by a lack of concentration and intermittent disorientation and agitated confusion. The latter is best treated with haloperidol 10 mg i.m. one-hourly as necessary (with a maximum of 60 mg/24 hour). This may precipitate dystonic reactions which may be relieved by benztropine 2 mg i.m.

(v) Promazine derivatives should not be used, because of their hepatotoxic effect, and opiates should be avoided as they may cause respiratory depression in persons with liver damage.

(vi) The possibility of cirrhosis, heart failure and neurological disease induced by alcohol should be considered during examination of the patient, as these may need treating also. To this end, the following investigations should be done as soon as possible: chest x-ray, ECG, liver function tests and serum proteins, Full blood picture and ESR, serum folate, electrolytes and blood urea.

(3) Remember all this is only first aid and your psychiatric colleagues should be involved as early as possible

The hypotensive patient[3,5,7]

DIAGNOSIS

A low arterial pressure reading *per se* does not matter unless there is also evidence of inadequate tissue perfusion, when it should always be regarded as a medical emergency. This combination also provides a working definition of shock. Poor tissue perfusion is most easily seen when it affects:

(1) The brain—mental confusion.
(2) The extremities (including the nose)—which are cold, pale, moist and mottled with peripheral cyanosis and collapsed veins.
(3) The kidneys—the minimal acceptable urine flow rate is 45 ml/hour. If it is less than this, renal hypoperfusion is likely to be present. If the temperature of the extremities falls much below that of the central temperature (as measured on a rectal thermometer) this implies poor tissue perfusion and a fall in the glomerular filtration rate is also likely.
(4) The coronary arteries—this may also be the cause of arrhythmias and also of impaired myocardial contractility.

The shock syndrome can arise from:

(1) Myocardial infarction (*see* p. 8) and/or heart failure from any cause.
(2) Pulmonary embolism (*see* p. 40).
(3) Cardiac arrhythmias—particularly Stokes-Adams attacks and ventricular tachycardias (*see* p. 17).
(4) Cardiac tamponade (*see* p. 51).
(5) Dissecting aneurysm (*see* p. 49).
(6) Salt and water depletion as in chronic renal failure (*see* p. 126), severe diarrhoea and vomiting, heat stroke and diabetic crisis.
(7) Haemorrhage (*see* p. 93).
(8) Mediastinal shift. This is usually due to massive pulmonary collapse (*see* p. 76), a large pleural effusion (*see* p. 81), over-hasty relief of a large pleural effusion (*see* p. 81) or a pneumothorax (*see* p. 73).
(9) Vasovagal attacks.
(10) Hypotensive therapy. This is usually mainly postural and may be exacerbated by salt and water depletion.

(11) Corticosteroid insufficiency (*see* p. 151).
(12) Circulating 'toxins', e.g. infarcted bowel (*see* p. 46), blood transfusion reactions (*see* below) or anaphylactic shock (*see* below).
(13) Drug overdosage (*see* p. 209).
(14) Acute gastric dilation (*see* p. 108).
(15) Extensive burns.

MANAGEMENT

Any of the above causes, if sufficiently prolonged or severe, may cause a reduced cardiac output and high peripheral resistance. The ensuing poor tissue perfusion causes a profound acidosis which dilates the precapillary arterioles, but not the post-capillary venules. This causes stagnation of blood within the capillaries which both exacerbates cellular hypoxia, and because of damage to the capillary walls, causes leakage of crystalloid and colloid from the vascular compartment. Further, in shock the entire capillary bed is involved, so that the capacitance of the vascular compartment is increased.

Thus, the initiating sequence of events in shock are compounded by:

(i)   Stasis of blood within the capillaries.
(ii)   Extravasation of crystalloid and colloid from damaged capillaries.
(iii) Increase in capacitance of the circulatory system.

The result of all this is a serious mis-match between the effective blood volume (much reduced) and the capacitance of the vascular compartment (increased). This mis-match is reflected clinically in the poor tissue perfusion, hypotension, tachycardia and lowered CVP which characterises shock. An understanding of these various factors is essential to the proper management of shock, which is further outlined below.

(1) Specific—directed towards removing the cause. This is, however, not usually sufficient, and further measures are required to correct tissue perfusion.
(2) Non-specific:

(i)   Restoring the circulating volume. Effective restoration of the circulating volume is the single most important measure in reversing shock. The questions to be answered are how much of which fluids will be required.

(a) How much? As outlined above, many factors contribute to the hypovolaemia of shock, and thus the volume of fluid required to restore perfusion is always greater than any fluid loss (which is, anyway, difficult to measure). Improving tissue perfusion is evidenced by a warming of the extremities, increasing renal flow and disappearance of mental confusion, and the amount of fluid to achieve this is best assessed by serial central venous pressure readings (*see* p. 277). A central venous pressure line is thus mandatory in the proper treatment of shock. Insertion of a Swan-Ganz catheter (*see* p. 281), enabling you to record pulmonary wedge pressure and cardiac output, can also be very helpful in assessing fluid requirements, and is being used more frequently in the monitoring of shock patients.

(b) Which fluids? Irrespective of the cause of shock, both crystalloids and colloids are lost, and both require replacement. The circumstances in which shock occurs will obviously determine the ratio of colloid to crystalloid used, but as a general rule, one-half to three-quarters of the necessary volume should be as crystalloid, and the rest as colloid. Crystalloids should be given initially as normal saline, as salt replacement has a first priority. However, in overall terms, there is usually more water than salt lost, and so it is reasonable to give one-third of the overall crystalloid replacement at 5% dextrose.

Colloid replacement can be as albumin, plasma or dextran. Dextran is cheap, readily available and free from the risk of hepatitis, and has, as an additional bonus, an anti-thrombotic property (*see* (vi) below). Dextran 70 in saline in a dose of 1000–1500 ml/24 hour, is widely regarded as the colloid of choice. If shock has been prolonged, dextran 40 which has the additional benefit of reducing viscosity, can be used in place of dextran 70. If colloid additional to the dextrans proves to be necessary, plasma may be used. In hypovolaemic cardiogenic shock, or in any other circumstances where saline infusion is undesirable dextran made up in dextrose can be used. Dextrans cause rouleaux formation, and so blood must be taken for cross-matching before they are infused. Haemocel, a colloid made from degraded gelatine, does not have anti-thrombotic properties. It does not cause cross-matching difficulties, but has no other advantages.

In haemorrhagic shock, blood will be required in addition to the above fluids. It is probably desirable to transfuse the patient to a haemoglobin of around 11 g/100 ml. Higher than this does not materially alter oxygen delivery, but does have the disadvantage of increasing viscosity.

(ii) Reversing hypoxia. Use of high (40–60%) concentrations of oxygen may improve the Pao$_2$ and will cause a small increase of oxygen in solution in the plasma. This may be sufficient to prevent some cell damage. This concentration can be achieved by most commercially available face masks using oxygen flow rates of about 10 l/min. Assisted ventilation may be required particularly if shock lung occurs (*see* p. 83). The use of hyperbaric oxygen is still experimental.

(iii) Reducing arteriolar constriction. This should be attempted if poor tissue perfusion persists despite adequate repletion of the circulatory volume.

It can be achieved either by:

(a) alpha-adrenergic blocking agents. These reduce arteriolar constriction. The agents most commonly used are phenoxybenzamine, phentolamine, chlorpromazine and nitroprusside. They can cause a disastrous fall in arterial pressure unless the expanded circulating volume is taken up by infusing fluid preferably blood, plasma or dextran 70 (molecular weight 70 000). It is essential for the central venous pressure to be at the upper limit of the normal range before these drugs are given. Infuse phenoxybenzamine 10–15 mg in 100 ml of 5% dextrose over 2 hours, or phentolamine at a rate of 0·5–1 mg/min or chlorpromazine 5 mg i.v. every 15 minutes to a maximum of 20 mg. Give nitroprusside as outlined on page 38. As the drug is given, the central venous pressure will probably fall together with the arterial pressure. The central venous pressure must be maintained within the upper half of the normal range by further infusions of fluid. This ensures an adequate venous return, and cardiac output.

or by:

(b) beta-adrenergic agents, e.g. isoprenaline. These also reduce arteriolar constriction and in addition have an inotropic effect on the heart. The arterial pressure of the hypotensive patient may be raised by increasing the cardiac output. Put 2 mg of isoprenaline in 500 ml of 5% dextrose and give the infusion sufficiently fast to raise the systolic arterial pressure to about 95 mmHg. If this is ineffective or leads to a large volume of fluid being infused, double or treble the concentration. Alternatively give dopamine (see p. 13). Both these are preferable to metaraminol (aramine) which has both alpha-mimetic and beta-mimetic properties and may increase the arterial pressure at some expense to tissue perfusion.

Noradrenaline and methoxamine should not be used. They constrict arterioles and further decrease tissue perfusion. Their use is therefore illogical, and in practice is rarely successful.

(iv) Glucocorticoids. In pharmacological doses they may have some inotropic effect on the heart, cause arteriolar dilation, and may protect against the development of shock-lung. Their role and action is not clear, and some do not favour their routine use.[9] However, we usually give sol-umedrone 2 g i.v. over 24 hours, or alternatively hydrocortisone 500 mg i.v. six-hourly for 6 doses. This sort of dose does not suppress the pituitary adrenal axis and so can be stopped abruptly.

(v) Increasing myocardial contractility. This can be achieved with adrenergic agents and with glucocorticoids as has already been mentioned. It may also be of benefit to digitalise the patient (see p. 34).

(vi) Reversing acidosis.[8] As acidosis has a well recognised negative inotropic effect, its correction is important, and is usually achieved by restoring tissue perfusion. However, if the pH is below 7·1 it is reasonable to give small quantities of bicarbonate. Theoretically the bicarbonate deficit (mmol) is given by (body weight (kg) × 3/5) × (25 – serum HCO_3 mmol/l). Give half this amount and repeat the arterial pH before deciding whether to give more.

(vii) More controversial is the use of heparin. Enzymes released from damaged cells convert fibrinogen to fibrin, thus creating a state of disseminated intravascular coagulation (DIC) which may further impair tissue perfusion. The evidence for DIC is a bleeding tendency with low platelets, raised prothrombic time (PT) and kaolin cephalin time (KCT), low fibrinogen titres and raised fibrin degradation products. These abnormalities are often reversed when the underlying cause of shock is corrected and there is no good evidence that the use of heparin increases survival.[11]

Blood transfusion reactions

A mild reaction consisting of flushing, itching and urticaria is quite common especially in those with a history of allergic reactions. Their incidence may be reduced by anti-histamines, e.g. diphenhydramine (Benadryl) 50 mg orally one hour before transfusion and 50 mg during it. If wheezing starts to occur or hypotension (which is not due to haemorrhage) develops, the blood should be stopped at once and saved for re-testing. Give hydrocortisone 200 mg i.v. or adrenaline 1:1000 0·5 ml subcutaneously immediately. Also give an intravenous anti-histamine such as diphenhydramine 20 mg i.v.

Acute renal failure as a complication of blood transfusion has been dealt with elsewhere (*see* p. 122).

Anaphylactic shock[4,6]

Never give any drug or vaccine to a patient who says he is allergic to it even if the evidence is unconvincing. Do not attempt to obtain the evidence by skin testing. This may be misleading and may occasionally be fatal. Warning signs are flushing, itching and urticaria. They may be absent. The symptoms of a more severe attack are wheezing, a feeling of chest constriction, abdominal pain, nausea and vomiting. Circulatory collapse and death may follow.

Give:

(1) Adrenaline 500–1000 μg (0·5–1·0 ml of 1:1000) i.m. to combat shock. This dose should be repeated at 15 minute intervals until improvement occurs.

(2) Diphenhydramine hydrochloride (Benadryl) 20 mg i.v. to counteract the excessive histamine release.

(3) Hydrocortisone 200 mg i.v. to suppress any further allergic reaction.

(4) Aminophylline 0·5 g i.v. over 5 minutes if there is evidence of continuing airways obstruction. Do not forget dyspnoea may also be due to acute laryngeal oedema (*see* p. 78).

(5) 35% oxygen if there is cyanosis.

(6) If there are signs of shock or if there is profound hypotension, establish a central venous pressure line and infuse plasma or dextran 70 or alternating bottles of normal saline and 5% dextrose to maintain a central venous pressure in the upper half of the normal range. This is usually sufficient to restore the arterial pressure. If, however, it remains low it may be necessary to give isoprenaline or dopamine (*see* p. 13).

Bacterial shock[13,14]

DIAGNOSIS

(1) Bacterial shock occurs when large numbers of bacteria get into the blood stream. Bacterial shock can be caused by both Gram +ve and Gram −ve organisms. Gram-negative organisms commonly spread after surgery to the bowel or instrumentation of the lower urinary tract. The organisms are usually *E. coli*, other coliforms, anaerobes or pseudomonas. Gram-positive organisms are often associated with joint and chest sepsis and drug abusage, and are usually staphylococci, streptococci or pneumococci. *Cl. welchii* septicaemia following abortion is an important special group (*see* Table III for antibiotic sensitivities (*see* p. 251).

(2) Whatever the organism the onset is usually marked by rigors associated with nausea, vomiting and diarrhoea. Initially the patient is peripherally vaso-dilated, flushed, pyrexial and hypotensive. Cardiac output is at this stage increased, but as much of the blood is being shunted through arterio-venous

communications, the $P\mathrm{ao}_2$ is low and tissue oxygen utilisation is deficient. The situation is peculiar to bacteraemic shock, and accounts for the paradox of an apparently well perfused patient who is, nonetheless, confused and oliguric. The mortality of this group is about 25%. This state gives way to the classical shock picture of a confused or comatose patient with cold, clammy peripheries, acidosis and a fall in urinary and cardiac output with or without pyrexia. The mortality of this group is at least 60%. Early recognition and energetic treatment of the former state may forestall the appearance of the latter with consequent saving of life.

MANAGEMENT

In about half the patients the interval between onset of shock and death is 48 hours, and a successful outcome is partially dependent upon the speed with which the following measures are carried out:

(1) Take blood for full blood count, electrolytes, urea and creatinine, group and cross-match, arterial blood gases and blood cultures. Do at least three blood cultures from different sites within half an hour. Take swabs from throat and rectum. Microscope and plate out a clean specimen of urine.

(2) Antibiotics. The initial drugs of choice are a combination of:

(i)   Gentamicin[16] which is bactericidal to most of the organisms commonly causing shock, except streptococci and anaerobes (i.e. Gram −ve rods such as bacteroides sp), and Gram +ve rods such as clostridium sp. Gentamicin is excreted unchanged in the urine and so dosage must be regulated in relation to renal function. With normal renal function toxicity rarely occurs at a dose of 5 mg/kg/day given in three divided doses. When renal function is impaired, the intervals between doses must be modified, (see Table II below); peak level (1 hour after i.v. or i.m. administration) should be between 8–15 μg/ml and trough levels (just before the next dose) should be around 2 μg/ml. Serum gentamicin levels should be monitored and the dosage modified accordingly.

An alternative way of calculating the dose interval is: serum creatinine (μmol/l) divided by 15 = approx. dosage

Table II **Modification of gentamicin dosage in patients with renal impairment**

Blood urea mmol/1	Dose and frequency of administration (for a 70 kg patient)
7	*80 mg h-hourly
7–18	*80 mg 12-hourly
18–36	*80 mg 24-hourly
36	*80 mg 48-hourly

*60 mg if patient is below 60 kg body weight

interval (in hours). This dose may range from 60 to 120 mg, depending on the weight of your patient.

The use of the newer aminoglycosides should be restricted to patients who are thought to have gentamicin resistance organisms. In these circumstances use either:

(a) Amikacin—15 mg/kg/day in two divided doses.
(b) Netilmicin—4–7 mg/kg/day in three divided doses.

Both these doses will have to be modified along the same lines as gentamicin if your patient has renal impairment.

(ii) Benzyl penicillin 2000 000 units six-hourly i.v. is effective against all streptococci and sensitive staphylococci. Many authorities also believe that given in combination with gentamicin, which suppresses penicillinase production, benzyl penicillin is effective against penicillinase producing organisms

(iii) If there has been recent pelvic or abdominal surgery, of if pus is reported by the laboratory as 'sterile' the likelihood of infection by anaerobes is high. In this case use in addition to (i) and (ii) above, either:

(a) Metronidazole—500 mg in 100 ml infused over half an hour, eight-hourly or 400 mg orally eight-hourly. This is the drug of choice.
(b) Clindamycin—300–600 mg i.v. six-hourly is highly effective but produces a severe pseudomembraneous colitis in a proportion of cases.

      (c) Chloramphenicol—(200 mg i.v. four-hourly) which is marginally less effective, but less toxic (the incidence of bone marrow suppression is extremely low in patients who have received less than 20 g of the drug).

or

      (d) Cephoxitin—this cephalosporin has a wide range of activity, and is effective against anaerobes. The dosage is 2 g six-hourly by i.v. infusion.

(iv) If overwhelming staphylococcal infection is suspected, 500 mg fucidin is dissolved in 250 cc of N saline and infused over 4 hours. Such an infusion is given 4 times/day.

(v) Azlocillin in a dose of 5 g eight-hourly i.v. can be used if pseudomonas infection is considered likely. It is synergistic with gentamicin but must be given in separate infusions, as they react chemically, inactivating each other. This reaction is only of serious consequence in the blood stream when renal function is seriously impaired. Fifteen grams of azlocillin includes 33 mmol of Na^+, and Na^+ administration should be adjusted accordingly.

(3) Fungal infection. Systemic candidiasis often occurs in the setting of a bacterial septicaemia. Remember a positive blood culture is not necessarily indicative of systemic disease, but if you believe there to be a significant candidal infection, the treatment is a combination of:

(i) Amphotericin B—first give a test dose of 1 mg in 20 ml 5% dextrose. Then, if no adverse reaction occurs, give 0·3 mg/kg on the first day and 0·6 mg/kg on subsequent days.

    Renal toxicity is a common problem after a few days therapy and you should temporarily stop the drug if the serum creatinine goes above 200 μmol/l.

and

(ii) Flucytosine—in a dose of 37·5 mg/kg/6 hours orally if renal function is normal. If the creatinine clearance is between 20 and 40 ml/min, reduce the dose interval to 12-hourly, and if it is 10–20 ml/min to 37·5 mg/kg each 24 hours.[14]

(iii) Miconazole—500–1000 mg i.v. can be used if amphotericin is contra-indicated.

Table III Table of sensitivity of common organisms to various antibiotics

	Staph. aureus Hosp	Staph. aureus Non-Hosp	Pseudomonas aeruginosa	E. coli	Proteus sp	Bacteroides sp	Clostridium welchi	Klebsiella aerobacter sp	Strep. pyogenes	Strep. faecalis
Azlocillin	R.	S.	S.S.	S.	S.	S.S.	H.S.	S.S.	S.	S.
Cephoxitin	S.	S.	R.	S.S.	S.	S.	S.	S.	S.	R.
Chloramphenicol	S.	S.	R.	S.	S.S.	S.	S.	S.	S.	S.
Gentamicin	H.S.	H.S.	S.	S.	S.	R.	R.	S.	R.	R.
Clindamicin	S.	S.	R.	R.	R.	H.S.	H.S.	R.	H.S.	R.
Benzyl Penicillin	R.	H.S.	R.	R.	R.	R.	H.S.	R.	H.S.	S.

Key: H.S. = Highly sensitive
S. = Sensitive
S.S. = Slightly sensitive
R. = Resistant

Clearly antibiotics to which organisms are either highly sensitive or sensitive should be used wherever possible.

(4) The restoration of tissue perfusion and correction of metabolic abnormalities are as detailed on p. 242, but:

(5) These patients are particularly prone to hypoxia, and frequently require assisted ventilation to maintain the $P\text{ao}_2$. This should be undertaken in conjunction with your anaesthetic colleagues. Even despite ventilatory assistance respiratory failure is a frequent mode of death. The lung capillaries appear to become leaky, giving an x-ray appearance of widespread consolidation. This respiratory complication is rather unsatisfactorily labelled shock lung (*see* p. 83).

(6) Naloxone. Endogenous opioids may be responsible for part of the initial hypotension in bacteraemic shock. Naloxone blocks the action of these endogenous opioids, and its role in shock is being evaluated. Preliminary evidence is that at a dose of 0·4–1·2 mg i.v. it may be useful.[15]

The unconscious patient

DIAGNOSIS

Coma is an unarousable lack of awareness. It is caused by the following:

(1) Bilateral and widespread dysfunction of both cerebral hemispheres.
(2) Damage to, or compression of, the activating centres of the brain stem and diencephalon.

} 33%

(3) Metabolic disturbance involving either of the above regions. It is to be distinguished from:

} 65%

(4) Psychogenic unresponsiveness.

} 2%

The pattern and sequencing of neurological abnormality can, to a large extent, distinguish which of these is most likely, thus providing information both as to localisation and cause. Since both these items are crucial to management, a careful history from relatives (or other witnesses, including the family practitioner or ambulance driver if necessary) and examination are mandatory.

WIDESPREAD DYSFUNCTION OF BOTH CEREBRAL HEMISPHERES

(1) Postictal stupor may, if a history is lacking, cause diagnostic confusion, which fortunately is temporary since the patient will usually rouse within 6 hours.
    Other causes are more serious and essentially are limited to:
(2) Catastrophic intra-cerebral or intra-ventricular haemorrhage (*see* p. 166).
(3) Closed head injury with contusion and/or intra-cerebral haemorrhage (*see* p. 174).

The picture of neurological disability here will depend upon the site of maximal involvement. Since each rapidly causes vasomotor paralysis, congestion and oedema of the brain with downward displacement of the cerebral hemispheres, the general effects are dealt with in the section immediately following.

INVOLVEMENT OF DIENCEPHALIC AND BRAIN-STEM ACTIVATING CENTRES

This may occur as the result of:

(1) **Pressure from expanding supratentorial mass lesions**. This implies evolution over time which, depending upon the rate of expansion, may vary from hours to weeks. This is likely to be the cause if there is a history of headache (other than occipital), head trauma, or preceding focal neurological signs or symptoms, or a strikingly asymmetrical neurological exam. The hallmark of this group is progressive involvement down the neuraxis—'rostral-caudal deterioration'. Expansion can impinge from two directions; these are discussed below.

(A) *Downwards—the central syndrome*. The early stages are marked by:

    (i)   Eupnoeic respirations which may be interrupted by sighs or yawns or by Cheyne-Stokes breathing.

    (ii)   Appropriately directed response to pain—for example, supra-orbital pressure.

    (iii) Paratonia 'gegenhalten'. Resistance to movement of a limb in any direction which is proportional to the force applied. This merges into increasing bilateral cortico-spinal and extra-pyramidal signs. Preceding hemiplegias become more marked. Sustained grasp reflexes—elicited by firm palmar pressure—emerge.

    (iv) Relative lack of brain stem involvement. Eye movements are intact, seen either spontaneously as rolling eye movements or in response to doll's head manoeuvre or ice water calorics which obtain ipsilateral *tonic* deviation of the eyes (without nystagmus). The doll's head manoeuvre is carried out by observing the effect on eye movements of briskly and fully rotating the head on the neck and trunk (if necessary whilst the patient is temporarily disconnected from the ventilator). Ice water calorics are carried out as follows. First, inspect the external auditory canal to ensure the tympanic membrane is intact and, if necessary, remove wax. Lift the head if possible to 30° to the horizontal. Using a thin catheter inserted into the external auditory canal, slowly instil up to 50 cc of ice cold water whilst observing the eye movements. In a conscious patient this is extremely uncomfortable for it induces severe vertigo, nausea and vomiting, together with nystagmus of which the fast component is away from the irrigated ear. In the unconscious patient with an intact brain stem, the response obtained is of *tonic* conjugate deviation of the eyes towards the irrigated ear. Having tested one side, 5 minutes should elapse before testing the other in order to allow the currents induced in the semicircular canals to subside. However, early posterior herniation through the tentorial incisura compresses the superior collicula and limits vertical eye movements (tested by briskly flexing the neck). The pupils are usually small, but careful exam with a bright light (and if necessary hand lens or ophthalmoscope) discloses an intact light reflex.

With further diencephalic compression, the directed response to pain is replaced by abnormal flexor posturing of the arms with extension of the legs—so-called 'decorticate' rigidity.

The importance of recognising this stage is that if the cause of the compression can be treated effectively—as, for example, oedema may—full recovery is likely. Further caudal involvement usually involves infarction, implying increasing morbidity and mortality (Table IV).

Involvement of the mid-brain and upper pons is signalled by:

(i)   Cheyne-Stokes respirations are replaced by tachypnoea.
(ii) Abnormal extensor postures of the arms with pronation of the forearms are evoked by pain—'decerebrate' rigidity.
(iii) The pupils dilate moderately to 3–5 mm and are frequently irregular.
(iv) Eye movements in response to doll's head manoeuvres and ice water calorics become harder to elicit. The adducting eye may fail to move past the mid position (internuclear ophthalmoplegia).

The lower pons—upper medulla stage—is reached when:

(i)   The respirations become shallow at 20–40 per minute;
(ii) The pupils stay at mid position (3–5 mm) but do not respond to light;
(iii) Eye movements become unobtainable;

Table IV Localisation of brain stem involvement

	Diencephalic			Mid brain	Lower pons	Lower medulla
	Upper		Lower			
	Central	Uncal		Upper pons	Upper medulla	
Response to pain	Appropriately directed	Appropriately directed	Abnormal flexor	Abnormal extensor	Nil	Nil
Pupils	Small with intact light reflex	Unilateral and then bilateral dilatation	Small with intact light reflex	3–5 mm irregular	3–5 mm and unresponsive	Dilated and unresponsive
Eye movements	Full (rolling)	Third nerve palsy	Full	Hard to elicit internuclear ophthalmoplegia	Absent	Absent
Respirations	Eupnoeic Cheyne-Stokes yawns	Eupnoeic	Eupnoeic	Tachypnoeic	Shallow 20–40 per minute	Slow and irregular
Other	Paratonia exacerbation of preceding deficits	Development of ipsilateral hemiplegia	—	Diabetes insipidus	—	Falling arterial pressure

(iv)   There is either no response to pain or occasionally a little leg flexion if the feet are stroked.

Terminally with medullary involvements:

(i)   The respiration slows and becomes irregular;
(ii)   The arterial pressure falls with a variably slow or fast heart rate.

(B) *From the side—uncal herniation.* This is usually caused by expanding masses in the lateral middle fossa (including the temporal lobe) which compresses the brain stem laterally. The diencephalon may be little involved initially; the third nerve almost invariably is. Thus, a unilaterally dilating pupil is accompanied by a level of consciousness which may vary from alertness to coma.

Once the pupil dilates fully, oculomotor involvement follows and ice water calorics reveal full third nerve impairment (failure of the eye to move from full abduction and downward deviation). All eye movement becomes lost as ischaemia spreads to the mid brain. Frequently the opposite cerebral peduncle becomes compressed against the tentorial edge, and a hemiplegia ipsilateral to the original lesion becomes added to the contra-lateral hemiplegia which frequently preceded it. Posturing in response to pain may be flexor but is usually extensor in the arm.

With involvement of the mid brain and upper pons, the opposite pupil may become fixed in mid position, and may also dilate widely. As with downward central compression, respiration becomes hyperpnoeic, extra-ocular movements become increasingly difficult to elicit and bilateral extensor posturing emerges.

(2) **Pressure may also arise from below with expanding subtentorial masses.** These may either be intrinsic to the brain stem, destroying the reticular activating system, or extrinsic, compressing it. Extrinsic lesions, in addition, may cause the cerebellum to herniate upwards through the tentorial notch, compressing the upper brain stem and diencephalon, and/or downwards through the foramen magnum, compressing the medulla.

The hallmark of this category of patients therefore is evidence of pontine or mid brain damage at the onset of coma. Further clues for a subtentorial lesion include a history of occipital headaches, vertigo, diplopia and/or vomiting at the onset of coma.

Initially therefore, before frank upward herniation, if there is compression of the middle third of the pons, the patient is usually drowsy rather than comatose, with constricted (1–2 mm) but reactive pupils and lateral rather than vertical ophthalmoplegia. Nystagmus—if present—is gaze paretic, respirations are initially unaffected but may later become ataxic and then slow; corticospinal tract signs and mild limb ataxia usually emerge.

As upward cerebellar herniation proceeds, signs of mid brain compression evolve with extensor posturing, unequal mid position fixed pupils with either failure of upward elevation of the eyes or frank downward conjugate deviation.

Downward herniation of the cerebellar tonsils may be suspected by resistance to neck flexion or spontaneous opisthotonic posturing, but if sufficiently advanced is obviously a terminal event, with respiratory and circulatory collapse ensuing shortly thereafter.

Destructive lesions within the brain stem are similarly accompanied by analogous brain stem signs depending on the site of maximal involvement. Typically the signs may be fairly restricted and frequently asymmetrical, thus providing accurate localisation. Thus:

(i)   Mid brain lesions, if centrally placed, interrupt the light reflex pathways and frequently interrupt oculomotor interconnections. Thus, pupils are mid position and fixed with either nuclear or internuclear (see above) ophthalmoplegia, and bilateral frequently asymmetrical corticospinal tract signs.

(ii) Rostral pons involvement is marked by small reactive pupils, internuclear ophthalmoplegia and sometimes evidence of fifth (absent corneal) or seventh (lower motor neuron facial asymmetry) nerve involvement.

(iii) Lower pons lesions similarly have small reactive pupils with lateral eye movements absent, but vertical eye movements spared (doll's head manoeuvre and ice water calorics). There may be a flaccid quadriplegia, or alternatively abnormal extensor posturing. The respiratory rhythm is frequently interrupted with cluster, apneustic or ataxic patterns.

If cerebellar and brain stem signs are elicited, the possibility of cerebellar haemorrhage (p. 170) must not be forgotten. Cerebellar infarcts accompanied by developing oedema may also behave like an expanding mass lesion and are similarly susceptible to potentially life-saving neurosurgical decompression.

METABOLIC ENCEPHALOPATHY

There are a number of features which distinguish this group of conditions from the preceding two categories.

(1) Coma is nearly always preceded by an interval of decreased awareness, impaired cognitive function and frequently personality disturbance.

(2) Even though other brain stem functions are lost with depression of consciousness, absent ice water caloric reflexes and abnormal extensor posturing, the pupillary light reflex is usually preserved. This simultaneous involvement of many levels of the neuraxis with relative sparing of some functions at the same level is typical of metabolic encephalopathy. Progressive rostral-caudal deterioration (*see* above) does not occur.

(3) Abnormal movements typical of metabolic encephalopathy include a fine tremor at 8–10 Hz, bilateral asterixis (frequently found in, but not confined to, hepatic encephalopathy) and multi-focal myoclonic jerks.

Sustained focal neurological deficits are usually absent. There are two exceptions to this rule which can be a trap, however:

(i) Hypoglycaemic hemiplegias which may completely resolve with prompt and adequate treatment (p. 146). Similar findings have been reported in hepatic coma, uraemia and hypernatraemia.

(ii) Although lateral conjugate deviation of the eyes strongly suggests a structural lesion, downward conjugate deviation may be caused by metabolic disturbance— particularly certain drug overdoses.

(4) Your examination will include smelling the breath (diabetic keto-acidosis, uraemic fetor, fetor hepaticus and alcohol) and testing for neck stiffness (meningitis, subarachnoid haemorrhage and tonsilar herniation).

PSYCHOGENIC UNRESPONSIVENESS

There are several features of this state which resolve diagnostic confusion:

(1) Eyelids are usually held firmly shut, resist opening, and when released snap shut. The slow passive closure of the lids of the comatose patient is rarely successfully reproduced.

(2) The corneal reflex evoked by blowing or by a wisp of cotton wool is rarely successfully suppressed. Similarly tickling the eyelashes usually evokes eyelid twitching.

(3) Roving or disconjugate eye movements exclude this diagnosis.

(4) Ice water calorics evoke nystagmus rather than tonic deviation.

MANAGEMENT

Evaluation of the evolution and patterns of neurological deficit should allow you to make a sophisticated guess at the site and nature of the lesion. However, common to all the categories are a number of basic considerations which in rough order or priority are:

(1) Assure oxygenation. This is quantified by measuring arterial gases or minute volume (more than 4 litres per minute). Clear secretions of blood and vomit by suction. If ventilation still seems inadequate intubate and ventilate. If there is a history of neck pain or trauma do not extend the neck to intubate. Obtain a lateral neck x-ray without moving the patient. Rarely an emergency tracheostomy may be necessary. Cardiac arrhythmias, provoked by intubation may be prevented by atropine 0·6 mg i.v. beforehand.

(2) Maintain circulation. If there is a vasomotor paresis from brain stem involvement or inadequate intake from prior illness, the effective circulating volume may be low. Infuse fluid in the usual way with CVP control (*see* p. 277). If the circulating volume is adequate, as judged by the CVP response, it may be necessary to infuse dopamine (*see* p. 13).

(3) Hypoglycaemia should be checked using B.M. stix, supplemented if reading low by a formal blood glucose. This should be done whilst (1) and (2) are going on.

(4) Fits. Other than brief minor motor episodes should be controlled (*see* p. 182).

(5) If there is evidence of a mass lesion (focal neurological signs

and/or signs of raised intra-cranial pressure) start treatment for raised intracranial pressure with a bolus of mannitol and controlled hyperventilation *see* p. 177). Obtain a CT scan; *do not* do a lumbar puncture.

(6) If there is evidence of metabolic disorder send blood for: (i) electrolytes and urea; (ii) osmolality; (iii) blood gases; (iv) calcium; (v) glucose. Save blood for toxic screen, liver function tests, coagulation studies, thyroid and adrenal function, blood culture and initial viral titre. If examining a traveller recently arrived from the tropics consider cerebral malaria, yellow fever, typhoid and typhus. Obtain a CT scan and in the absence of focal swelling do a lumbar puncture.

(7) Check the rectal temperature. Extremes of temperature should be corrected (*see* p. 229).

(8) If there is a history of alcoholism, or if there is ophthalmoplegia, or if the intravenous dextrose is ιo be infused, give thiamine 100 mg i.v. beforehand to prevent or treat Wernickes encephalopathy.

(9) If you suspect a narcotic overdose give naloxone 0·4 mg every 5 minutes until the patient arouses. If there is evidence of narcotic addiction (look for needle marks), dilute 0·4 mg in 10 cc of diluent and inject slowly to avoid precipitating an acute withdrawal crisis.

(10) If coma is interrupted by agitation, small (5 mg), preferably intravenous, doses of diazepam should suffice.

(11) General care of the unconscious patient includes:

(i) Attention to pressure points (a pillow between the arms, two-hourly turning, perhaps a ripple mattress). Obviously bed linen must be frequently changed if it becomes soaked with urine or stained with faeces.

(ii) In the absence of spontaneous blinking avoid exposure keratitis by methylcellulose eye drops and, if necessary, securing the eyelids with adhesive tape.

(iii) Urinary incontinence can frequently be managed satisfactorily with a sheath urinal for a man, but for women an indwelling silastic catheter inserted with strict attention to asepsis is the most satisfactory solution.

Severe chest pain[21]

DIAGNOSIS

Consider:

(1) **The heart**
Angina.
Myocardial infarction (*see* p. 8).
Cardiac arrhythmias (*see* p. 17).
Pericarditis—the pain is often affected by posture, and is usually worse lying down. It is also promptly relieved by indomethacin.

(2) **The lungs**
Pneumonia (*see* p. 86) and other causes of pleurisy.
Pulmonary embolus (*see* p. 40).
Pneumothorax (*see* p. 73).
Carcinoma of the lung.

(3) **The oesophagus**
Oesophagitis, with or without hiatus hernia.
Oesophageal achalasia.
Ruptured oesophagus—this gives rise to mediastinal emphysema, thus you may feel crepitus at the root of the neck.
Oesophageal carcinoma.

(4) **The aorta**
Dissecting aneurysm (*see* p. 49).

(5) **The mediastinum**
Mediastinitis.
Mediastinal pneumothorax.

(6) **The nerves**
Cervical spondylitis or other causes of root compression.
Herpes zoster—you will be vindicated should a characteristic rash appear.

(7) **The abdomen**
Acute cholecyctitis.
Acute exacerbation or perforation of a peptic ulcer.
Pancreatitis.

(8) **Thoracic wall**
An almost endless list of conditions involving muscles, bones, nerves, etc.—of which perhaps the commonest is an unexplained sharp pain over the precordium, lasting a few moments, called 'precordial catch'.

MANAGEMENT

The possibilities can usually be reduced to two or three by a careful history and examination.

However, it is wise always to ask for:

(1) An ECG.
(2) A chest x-ray.

And if in doubt, observe the patient in hospital, bearing in mind that a normal ECG does not exclude a myocardial infarction.

Severe headaches

The commonest cause of severe headache is migraine. Usually there is a preceding history of episodic throbbing headaches associated with nausea and photophobia. Classically, visual symptoms such as teichopsia, fortification spectra, etc., may precede or accompany the headache. Neck stiffness from concomitant muscle spasms, photophobia, and transient focal signs (*see* p. 171) may mimic meningitis which must, in cases of doubt, be excluded by examination of the CSF.

Causes which are emergencies are:

(1) A. Meningitis.[24] This has four cardinal signs: headache, stiff neck, photophobia and fever. They may be all absent. A lumbar puncture is indicated if two of the four are present. It may also present itself as drowsiness, confusion, convulsions, focal neurological signs or coma. In the immunologically uncompromised host three organisms account for most cases of bacterial meningitis. These are *Neisseria meningitidis* (usually affecting young adults), *Haemophilus influenzae* (usually in the under fives) and *Streptococcus pneumoniae* (any age group, and the prominent organism in the elderly).

The organism may be identified by direct staining of CSF. However, where no organisms can be seen, for example, in partially treated meningitis, distinguishing antigens may rapidly be identified after counterimmune electrophoresis, until positive identification is secure give either:

  (i) Benzyl penicillin 250 000 units/kg/day in divided doses at four-hourly intervals and chloramphenicol 100 mg/kg/day i.v. in divided doses at six-hourly intervals; or

  (ii) Cefuroxime 3 g eight-hourly (children 60–75 mg/kg eight-hourly)[28]

When the organism is identified proceed as follows:

  (i) *Neisseria meningitidis*—meningococcal meningitis, benzyl penicillin is the drug of choice given as above. If intravenous therapy becomes technically difficult and the organism is sensitive to sulphonamides these may be given orally instead.

(ii) *Streptococcus pneumoniae*—pneumococcal meningitis. Again give benzyl penicillin as above.

(iii) *Haemophilus influenzae*. Chloramphenicol is once again the drug of choice. Previously ampicillin 300 mg/kg/day i.v. in divided doses given six-hourly was advocated. This has now been precluded by the rapid rise in incidence of ampicillin resistance.

Patients with pyogenic meningitis who are allergic to penicillin or in whom the organism has not been identified should be given chloramphenicol as above. Triple therapy with penicillin, sulphonamide, and chloramphenicol, intrathecal antibiotics, and steroids are unnecessary in treating meningitis caused by these organisms.

Differentiation from other causes of meningitis rests on examination and culture of the CSF:

(1) B. Tuberculous meningitis. This may present itself with a few weeks history of increasing headaches, malaise and drowsiness, or have a more acute course of seizures, focal signs and progressive obtundation. Evidence of tuberculous infection elsewhere may be lacking but the tuberculin skin test is usually positive. All cases of suspected meningitis should have CSF examined and cultured for TB organisms since although the CSF cell response is typically lymphocytic, occasionally polymorphs may predominate. Recommended therapy is isoniazid 10–15 mg/kg/day (plus pyridoxine 50 mg/day) with rifampicin 600 mg/day and either ethambutol 25 mg/kg/day or pyrazinamide (0·5 g t.i.d., p.o.). Cryptococcal meningitis is not uncommon in America and is not confined to the diabetic or otherwise immunologically compromised. History is similar to that for tuberculous meningitis and likewise may be acute or more insidious. Diagnosis is made by India ink microscopy of the CSF and examination for cryptococcal antigens. Recommended therapy is a combination of amphotericin and flucytosine, in the same dosage as for candidal septicaemia (*see* p. 250).

Amoebic meningitis is usually identified only when pyogenic meningitis fails to respond to conventional therapy since the amoeba in CSF resembles white cells. Recommended therapy is amphotericin B 20 mg/day or if the organism is a hartmanella species sulphadiazine 100 mg/kg/day given as six-hourly doses i.v.

Unusual organisms may cause meningitis in immunologically compromised people. The treatment of these is beyond the scope of this book.

(2) Sub-arachnoid haemorrhage (*see* p. 166).
(3) Giant cell arteritis.[22, 23]

This condition commonly causes headache by involvement of the medium sized arteries of the scalp or dura and is virtually unheard of below the age of 55 years. In about half the cases involvement of the central retinal artery causes blindness which usually occurs between one and three months after the onset of the headaches. However, transient or permanent amblyopia may be the presenting symptom. In the typical case the superficial arteries are tender, swollen and often pulseless. The ESR is frequently more than 60 mm in the first hour. Occasionally superficial arteries are not clinically involved and the ESR is normal. Where the history is suggestive a length of temporal artery when examined serially may show the characteristic histology. High doses of steroids, e.g. 60 mg of prednisone per day should be given immediately the diagnosis is suspected.

(4) Hypertensive encephalopathy (*see* p. 37).
(5) Herpes encephalitis. Here the headache is accompanied by a 3–4 day course of increased irritability, confusion, neck stiffness and in the later stages occasional seizures followed by progressive stupor. Percussion of the skull may demonstrate lateralised tenderness. CSF shows lymphocytosis, raised protein count and characteristically increased red cells. Typically temporal lobe involvement may be demonstrated by EEG, radionucleide scan and a little later by CT scan. However, herpes encephalitis may be more generalised or focal elsewhere. Herpes simplex vesicles are rarely found on lips, skin or genitalia but where present virions may be identified by electron microscopy of vesicle fluid. Failing this the brain should be biopsied at the site of maximum involvement and sent for culture. The need for haste and accurate diagnosis rests on one controlled trial demonstrating the effect of adenosine arabinoside.[27] Mortality was apparently reduced by this drug given as 15 mg/kg/day in a 12-hour i.v. infusion for 10 days. The authors' experience of this drug has been disappointing. However, Acyclovir which has a similar mode of action but is more potent has been more clinically impressive in our hands. We advocate using 5 mg/kg i.v. eight-hourly for 5 days.

(6) Subdural haematoma (*see* p. 167).
(7) Pituitary apoplexy (*see* p. 149).

The acutely breathless patient

Consider:

(1) Left ventricular failure (*see* p. 32).
(2) Pulmonary embolus (*see* p. 40).
(3) Mitral stenosis (*see* p. 34).
(4) Cardiac tamponade (*see* p. 51).
(5) Asthma (*see* p. 69).
(6) Acute respiratory tract infections (*see* p. 62).
(7) Pneumothorax (*see* p. 73).
(8) Large pleural effusion (*see* p. 81).
(9) Acute upper airways obstruction (*see* p. 78).
(10) Massive pulmonary collapse (*see* p. 76).
(11) Myasthenia (*see* p. 189).
(12) Acute infective polyneuritis (*see* p. 186).
(13) Overdose of salicylates, dinitrophenol or sulphanilamide (*see* p. 213).
(14) Overbreathing ostensibly due to anxiety (often called 'hysterical' overventilation).

OVERBREATHING DUE TO ANXIETY

(1) This usually occurs in young women. The overbreathing may be far from obvious to the casual observer.
(2) The history is nearly always classical; first they felt breathless— then they had tingling, first round the mouth, then in the arms and legs; then they had cramps of the hands which took up the main d'accoucheur position. If sufficiently prolonged the patient may lose consciousness.
(3) You must aim to establish the sequence of events. In this condition anxiety precedes breathlessness, whereas in the other causes of breathlessness, the converse is usually the case.
(4) Emergency treatment is to persuade the patient to breathe in and out of a paper bag. This allows them to rebreathe their CO_2, lower the pH, reverse the alkalosis and relieve the tetany. This relieves most of the tension and is accompanied by massive verbal reassurance and, if necessary, sedation with 50 mg of chlorpromazine or 10 mg diazepam.

(5) Do not leave it at that—try and establish the precipitating cause. Their anxiety may be due to a somatic or psychiatric condition for which they may need help.

(6) Do not forget that anxious overbreathing young women may also have taken an overdose of salicylates. Always test the urine.

In other states such as diabetic ketosis, the uraemic syndrome, and encephalitis, the patient is obviously breathing abnormally deeply—but this is rarely attended by the distress which accompanies the above conditions.

Social problems

Some people who arrive at casualty departments turn out to be unable to provide for themselves and are often referred to the medical team.

They include:

(1) (i)   the frail elderly patient who does not require admission on strictly medical grounds;

    (ii)   the patient who comes to casualty with a trivial illness, but is of no fixed abode;

    (iii) the mother who, as a result of contracting a minor illness is unable to cope at home because of poor circumstances and innumerable children;

    (iv) the psychiatric patient who needs in-patient treatment, but will not come in.

(2) The basic requirements enabling an individual to fend for himself are:

    (i)   food;

    (ii)   money;

    (iii) shelter and clothes;

    (iv) companionship—in its widest sense;

    (v)   mental stability (to the extent that they will neither harm themselves or other people) and the ability to manage (i) to (iv).

Help to provide for these requirements may be forthcoming from:

(1) Your hospital social worker who should always be contacted first if possible. If you do not have one, or the problem arises at night and the social worker is unavailable:

(2) Your local authority Social Services Department who should provide a 24-hour social work service. Ring their duty officer for advice on:

    (i)   Psychiatric problems. It is clearly wise to avail yourself of any local psychiatric help first, either within your hospital, or from the area mental hospital, but this may not always be forthcoming. In any case you may need a social worker

to help you to commit a patient against his will to hospital under the appropriate section of the Mental Health Act.
   (ii)   Problems with children. Your hospital may provide facilities for admitting young children with their mother— if not, it may be necessary that they be taken into care via the Social Services Department.
   (iii) The elderly. If the advice of a geriatrician is not easily available social work advice re domiciliary services and/or residential accommodation is essential.

(3) Many areas have hostels either run by the Department of Health and Social Security (DHSS), Social Services, or voluntary organisations, e.g. The Salvation Army, for people of no fixed abode. Your casualty department has the telephone number of these hostels, which, however, are under no obligation to take people. The DHSS should provide for each area an emergency office which is open in the evenings for emergency payments or provision of hostel vouchers.
(4) The patient's General Practitioner (if he has one) who will be able to provide valuable background information and should be contacted, if available.
(5) Voluntary organisations, e.g. The Samaritans who provide a 24-hour supportive service for those in acute distress; e.g. suicides, or other similar organisations (e.g. Alcoholics Anonymous, Depressives Anonymous, Gingerbread (mainly daytime)).
(6) The police who carry place of safety warrants (for children and the mentally ill) and are a source of information re local hostels.

If these organisations cannot immediately help, the person should be admitted to hospital *pro tem*.

SECTION X REFERENCES

Alcohol withdrawal

1   Hollister LE, Prusmack JJ, Lipscomb W. Treatment of acute alcohol withdrawal with chlormethiazole. *Diseases of the nervous system* 1972; **33**: 247.
2   Leader. Management of alcohol withdrawal symptoms. *Br Med J* 1981; **1**: 502.

Hypotensive patient

3   Allison JP. Metabolic aspects of intensive care. *Br J Hosp Med* 1974; **11**: 860.
4   Austen KF. Systemic anaphylaxis in the human being. *N Engl J Med* 1974; **291**: 66.
5   Gruber UF. Hypovolaemic shock—therapy of hypovolaemic and respiratory insufficiency. *Triangle* 1974; **13**: No 3, 91.
6   Leader. Treatment of anaphylactic shock. *Br Med J* 1981; **1**: 1011.
7   Joseph SP. The management of acute hypotension. *Br J Hosp Med* 1976; **16**: 349.
8   Wassirer JP. Serious acid base disorder. *N Engl J Med* 1974; **291**: 773.
9   Sheagren JN. Septic shock and corticosteroids. *N Engl J Med* 1981; **305**: 456.
10 Garrod LP, Lambert HP, O'Grady F. *Antibiotics and chemotherapy, 280*. London: Churchill Livingstone, 1973.

Bacterial shock

11 Bergentz SE. Septic shock and disturbances in coagulation. *Triangle*; **13**: No 3, 129.
12 Cartwright RV. Antifungals. *Br Med J* 1978; **2**: 108.
13 Ledingham L McA. Prospective study of the treatment of septic shock. *Lancet* 1978; **1**: 1194.
14 Editorial. Bacteraemic shock. *Lancet* 1974; **1**: 296.
15 Editorial. Naloxone for septic shock. *Lancet* 1981; **1**: 38.
16 Noone P. Aminoglycosides. *Br Med J* 1978; **2**: 549.
17 Cohen J. Antifungal chemotherapy. *Lancet* 1982; **2**: 532.

271

Coma and care of unconscious/paralysed patient

18   England EJ. Intermittent catheterisation of the paralysed bladder. *Br J Urology* 1972; **44**: 278.
19   Sabin TD. The differential diagnosis of coma. *N Engl J Med* 1974; **290**: 1062.
20   Plum F, Posner JB. The diagnosis of stupor and coma. Philadelphia: FA Davis, 1982.

Chest pain

21   Lichstein E, Seckler SG. Evaluation of acute chest pain. *Med Clin North Am* 1973; **57**: 1481.

Severe headaches

22   Cullen JF. Ophthalmic complications of giant cell arteritis. *Surv Ophthalmol* 1976; **20**: 247.
23   Klein RG, Campbell RJ, Hunder GG, *et al.* Skip lesion in temporal arteritis. *Mayo Clin Proc* 1976; **51**: 504.
24   Lambert HP. Meningitis. *Br Med J* 1978; **2**: 259.
25   Johansson O. Cefuroxime versus ampicillin and chloramphenicol for the treatment of bacterial meningitis. *Lancet* 1982; **1**: 295.
26   Seligman JJ. The rapid differential diagnosis of meningitis. *Med Clin Nth Am* 1973; **6**: 1417.
27   Whitley RJ, Soong SJ, Dolin R. Adenine arabinoside therapy of biopsy-proven herpes simplex encephalitis. *N Engl J Med* 1977; **297**: 289.
28   Swedish Study Group. Cefuroxime versus ampicillin and chloramphenicol for the treatment of bacterial meningitis. *Lancet* 1982; **1**: 295.

CENTRAL VENOUS PRESSURE AND SWAN-GANZ CATHETER

Central venous pressure[1,2,5]

CVP measurements play an important role in many medical emergencies. This is now a standard technique in which careful attention to detail is necessary for reliable results to be obtained.

TECHNIQUE[1]

Your objective is to introduce an intravenous catheter into the superior vena cava. So introduce an intravenous catheter into a vein which will give you ready access to the superior vena cava. This is preferably done percutaneously or if necessary by cutting down on the vein and introducing the catheter under direct vision. The vein most often used is the median cubital or basilic vein, though any vein which has ready access to the superior vena cava may be used; for example, the external or internal jugular or sub-clavian.

Difficulty may be experienced negotiating the section of the basilic vein where it passes under the clavi-pectoral fascia. It may be over-come by twisting the catheter so that its natural lie is in the line of the vein, by abducting the arm to a right angle and externally rotating it, or by passing the catheter onwards while at the same time infusing fluid through it, thus displacing the walls of the vein. The position of the catheter MUST be checked after insertion by x-ray. If it is in the superior vena cava the level should rise and fall a few millimetres with expiration and inspiration. If it does not:

(i)   it is not in a vein;
(ii)   you are not far enough up the vein;
(iii) the tip is angled against the vein wall—withdraw slightly;
(iv)   the catheter is partially blocked—flush out with 5 ml of sodium citrate;
(v)   the catheter tip is in the right ventricle—the level is sus-piciously high and pulsatile.

The catheter is connected by a three-way stopcock to a water man-ometer. The scale should be zeroed against a fixed reference point on the patient who should, therefore, always be in the same position when the measurements are taken. The following values all apply to the horizontal patient lying supine:

Reference point	*Normal values*
5 cm dorsal from angle of Louis	1 to 8 cm
The angle of Louis	−4 to +3 cm

The reference point of 10 cm above the surface on which the patient is lying is not acceptable.

INTERPRETATION

The measurement obtained reflects at least four variables:

- (i)   intrathoracic pressure;
- (ii)   efficiency of the right heart;
- (iii) venous tone; and
- (iv)   volume of venous blood.

It may appear surprising, therefore, that useful results can be obtained at all. These variables are examined in more detail below.

- (i)   The gentle oscillation associated with respiration which was noted above, reflects change in the intrathoracic pressure.
- (ii)   The efficiency of the right heart should not be compromised unless the circulation is being overloaded or there is myocardial disease. However, it is vital to remember that the CVP measures right atrial pressure and often fails to reflect left atrial pressure, particularly in the presence of myocardial disease. In these circumstances a patient may develop severe left ventricular failure without altering the CVP and a pulmonary artery pressure line (with facilities for measuring pulmonary wedge pressure) should be set up wherever this is available (*see* p. 9).
- (iii) The fact that venous tone cannot be measured in the clinical situation neither refutes its existence nor diminishes its importance. The capacitance of the circulation is controlled by venous tone, which is therefore a primary influence upon CVP as a measure of the volume of venous blood. Venous tone is increased for instance by both catecholamine infusion and haemorrhagic shock. In these clinical circumstances, a relatively high CVP may be more a reflection of raised venous tone than adequate blood volume.

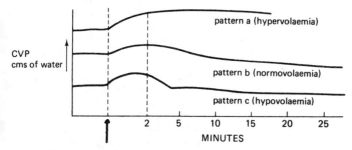

CVP
cms of water

BOLUS INFUSION OF 200 mls OF FLUID

Fig. 24.

(iv) In normal circumstances the venous system is readily dis-
      tensible; venous tone may relax to the extent that a sub-
      stantial increase of blood volume may produce no change
      in CVP. For these reasons a single recording of CVP is
      unlikely to be helpful in assessing and monitoring the
      replacement of blood volume. A series of readings is more
      likely to be informative, particularly if they are taken in
      response to rapid but small increments in blood volume.
      Specifically, if 200 ml of fluid is infused over 2 minutes, we
      recognise three patterns of response (*see* Fig. 24):

      (a) a persistent rise of more than 3 cm of water can be
           taken to exclude hypovolaemia and probably implies
           hypervolaemia (pattern a);
      (b) a rise of 2–3 cm during the infusion with return to the
           base line at 15–20 minutes is characteristic of nor-
           movolaemia (pattern b);
      (c) a rise of 2–3 cm during the infusion with return to the
           base line within 5 minutes is highly suggestive of
           hypovolaemia (pattern c).

           An initial reading of the CVP which is well within
      the normal range should not put you off performing
      this diagnostic/therapeutic test because as mentioned
      above, a high venous tone may raise the CVP and mask
      hypovolaemia. If hypovolaemia is suspected on clinical
      grounds careful expansion of the circulating volume
      with the CVP maintained a few cm above normal (but

less than 10 cm above the angle of Louis, otherwise pulmonary oedema may be precipitated) should be tried. For details of which fluids to infuse see p. 243. This may actually cause a slow fall of central venous pressure by inducing relaxation of the veins and allow infusion of more fluid. This gradual fall in CVP may also be observed in response to both vasodilators and steroids, or if an infusion of pressor amines is stopped. Where hypovolaemia has been confirmed, infuse fluid rapidly until the CVP rises into the upper half of the normal range. If this level is maintained for several hours the patient will become warmer and pinker, and will start to look better. A satisfactory urine output may also be restored (but be on your guard for acute renal failure) (see p. 124). It is now reasonable to run the infusion at a normal rate and allow the CVP to fall. Should the CVP drop below normal, full fluid repletion has not taken place and an infusion rate sufficient to keep the CVP in the mid-normal range is required. The deleterious effects of hypovolaemia are due to poor tissue perfusion. Although a low cardiac output is usually the primary cause of poor perfusion, the subsequent hypoxia produces locally and centrally mediated responses in the peripheral vasculature which aggravate the situation (see p. 242). Typically there is (a) arteriolar constriction producing a further reduction in tissue flow, and (b) venular dilatation which pools blood in the periphery reducing venous return and therefore cardiac output. Clearly the longer a patient remains hypovolaemic the more firmly this vicious circle becomes established. For this reason the consequences of prolonged hypovolaemia can only be reversed by maintaining the CVP within or above the upper range of normal for several hours. Large volumes of up to 15–20 litres may be required and can only be given safely with a reliable CVP line. Any excess of water and electrolytes may be excreted after normal homeostasis has been restored without harmful effects.

OTHER USES

(1) In conditions where the problem concerns myocardial efficiency rather than hypovolaemia (e.g. myocardial infarction) a rise in CVP may give warning of impending heart failure. Remember that in these circumstances the CVP may not reflect left ventricular function, and that in any case a CVP line is no more than a jugular venous pulse with a college education.

(2) A sudden fall in the central venous pressure in a patient with suspected gastro-intestinal bleeding may herald further blood loss before this becomes clinically apparent (*see* p. 95).

(3) Prolonged intravenous feeding is only possible through a central venous pressure line.

(4) Blood samples may be withdrawn through a central venous pressure line providing 20 ml is withdrawn first (and of course rejected) to clear the dead space.

COMPLICATIONS

Although CVP measurements are of enormous help in situations of hypovolaemia and to a lesser extent myocardial infarction, venous catheters may be associated with complications and they should not therefore be used unless a definite therapeutic advantage is expected. The following complications have all been recorded.

(1) Thrombophlebitis. This is almost inevitable if the catheter is left in for more than 10 days and is probably due to mechanical irritation. The inflammation is rapidly settled by short-wave therapy but a blocked vein is inevitable and occasionally oedema of the upper arm results.

(2) Infection of the cut-down site.[4] This is minimised by scrupulous aseptic technique and polybactrin spray. It is also a good idea to separate the sites of entry of the catheter through the skin and into the vein as far as possible.

(3) Infection of the catheter tip is less easily avoided and may give rise to septicaemia. At any rate, it is a wise precaution to culture the catheter tip after it has been removed.

(4) Erosion of the vein. If this is not recognised early it may cause widespread infusion of fluid into subcutaneous tissues, which is painful for the patient and may be dangerous if secondary infection occurs. If suspected, the catheter should be withdrawn.

(5) Arterial bleeding sufficient to cause tracheal obstruction is a potential complication of all jugular and subclavian puncture techniques.

(6) Pneumothorax is a specific complication of subclavian vein puncture.

(7) Catheter embolus into the right heart is known to occur if the catheter is inadvertently broken at the site of entry to the skin. Surgical advice should be sought.

The Swan-Ganz catheter[3]

Pulmonary wedge pressure

Knowledge of the left and right atrial pressures is essential for the informed management of complicated acute heart failure. It is also wise to have an arterial cannula for continuous monitoring of pressure and for blood gas analysis. Finally, cardiac output measurement, perhaps something of a luxury, provides all the information necessary to manage the most complex haemodynamic problems.

The Swan-Ganz catheter

Right atrial pressure is measured with a CVP line (*see* p. 276), whilst left atrial pressure is most conveniently measured using a flow directed pulmonary artery catheter (Swan-Ganz catheter). This can be put in at the bedside without x-ray control. The left atrial pressure at which pulmonary oedema will appear is dependent on the serum albumin. A simple formula expresses this dependence (*see* p. 32).

(A) The catheter

Has two lumens, one of which controls a balloon immediately behind the catheter tip, whilst the other opens as a single end-hole. The balloon has a dual function; during insertion it is blown-up (with air or CO_2) as soon as the catheter tip is in a central vein. Thereafter the balloon acts as a sail, directing the catheter tip in the direction of maximal flow, i.e. through the tricuspid and pulmonary valves. Once the tip is in a small pulmonary artery, inflation of the balloon will occlude the artery proximally, leaving the end-hold exposed to the pulmonary capillary pressure (pulmonary wedge pressure), which is assumed to be identical with left atrial pressure.

Swan-Ganz catheters are usually available in two sizes:

7F with a 1·5cc balloon
5F with a 0·8cc balloon

We have found the larger size easier to manipulate and less likely to clot. For cardiac output measurement, using the thermodilution technique, catheters are available with an additional injection lumen in the right atrium and two thermistors beyond.

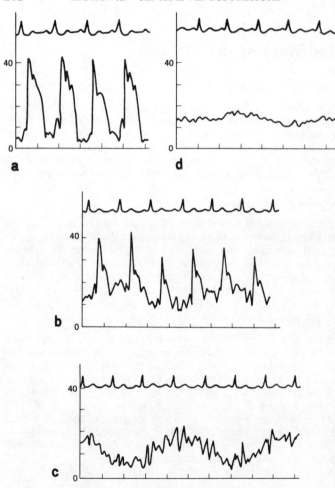

Fig. 25. Pressure tracings from the right heart. (a) Right ventricle; (b) Pulmonary artery; (c) Pulmonary artery wedge pressure; (d) Damped wedge pressure tracing. The pressure scale is in mmHg. The paper speed is 25 mm/sec with 10 mm spaces shown. The base line variation in the tracings is due to the effect of respiration. An ECG recording is also displayed.

(B) Catheter insertions

This is best by an antecubital cut down on the basilic vein—a technique free of serious complications. Alternatively the catheter can be put into a large central vessel percutaneously. 7F catheters require a guide-wire technique; we use DESSELET insertion sheaths. Remember to use a sheath *one size larger* than the catheter to allow for the deflated balloon. 5F catheters can be passed through large cannulae, e.g. a 12.G. medicut, but a guide-wire technique is probably safer.

(1) Advance the catheter into the vein—say 10 cm—and connect to the transducer (*see* Measurement below).

(2) Blow up the balloon when the tip is in a central vein.

(3) Advance slowly allowing the catheter tip to be guided by flow. Except in conditions of very low flow, it is usually easy to cross the valves. If there is trouble crossing the pulmonary valve it is worth trying the balloon both deflated and inflated to get across. Sometimes loops form in the right atrium which make manipulation difficult. Withdraw the catheter with the balloon blown up in order to straighten it out.

(4) Try to find a position which gives a good pulmonary artery tracing with the balloon deflated (Fig. 25 (b)) and a good wedge pressure with it inflated (Fig. 25 (c)). The right ventricular pressure tracing (Fig. 25 (a)) is shown for comparison.

(5) x-ray the chest.

(C) Measurement

The exact set-up will vary with the equipment available. Most equipment designed for continuous monitoring is pre-calibrated such that a given pressure change produces a set deflection on the scale. It therefore only remains to zero the transducer to atmospheric pressure. Some equipment may require both zero and calibration adjustment in which case it is necessary to adjust the calibration using a mercury column.

(1) The catheter is connected via a manometer line, a three-way tap and an INTRAFLO continuous flushing device to the transducer. The INTRAFLO is also connected to a pressure bag containing N saline and 500 units heparin.

(2) As the transducer is set up exclude all air bubbles from the system.

(3) To zero the transducer:

    (i)   close the tap between catheter and transducer (if this is not done, blood will flow back up the catheter into the transducer dome);

    (ii)   open the tap on the side arm of the transducer to air;

    (iii)   adjust the tracing on the monitor to zero;

    (iv)   close the transducer side arm and open the transducer to the catheter. Zero the transducer after it has warmed up—this will take about 30 minutes. Remember that the wave form used for catheter positioning does not have to be quantitatively accurate; we ordinarily put the catheter in first and then zero (and calibrate if necessary) afterwards.

(4) Recordings are made

    (i)   with the patient flat;

    (ii)   with the transducer at the level of the angle of Louis or mid chest (*see* CVP p. 000). This is most important;

    (iii)   of phasic and then mean pulmonary wedge pressure. The phasic nature of the recording is due to the pressure swings related to respiration, and it is the mean pulmonary wedge pressure which you should act on. (Many monitors produce a digital display of systolic, diastolic and mean pressures.)

(5) Before acting on a single or serial recording, it is essential to check their validitiy. Check:

    (i)   transducer level;

    (ii)   zero;

    (iii)   that there is no 'over wedging' (*see* below).

If you have any reason to disbelieve the calibration of a preset machine, it is easy to attach a manometer line to the transducer side arm and produce a vertical column of water. (13·5 cm H_2O = 10 mmHg.) Important decisions may be made on the basis of differences of less than 4 mmHg in the wedge pressure, that is 20% of the upper limit of normal. It is easy to make errors of this order in recording.

(D) Problems

(1) 'Over-wedging'. Sometimes the catheter tip is lodged in a small

pulmonary artery whose diameter is less than that of the balloon. As the balloon is blown up a wedge tracing appears and starts climbing continuously. If this happens, fill the balloon slowly, stopping as soon as the wedge appears. Make sure the trace rises and falls with respiration.

(2) Failure to wedge. Try repositioning the catheter. Alternatively, pulmonary artery diastolic pressure usually approximates to wedge pressure.

(3) Damped trace (Fig. 25 (d)) and blocked catheters. This is the major problem with continuous monitoring.

    (i)   check that there is no air in the system and that the transducer is not open both to air and to the patient;

    (ii) try flushing the catheter using the fast flush mechanism on the INTRAFLO;

    (iii) try a hand flush. Use a 1 ml syringe—being of narrow bore this generates the highest pressures. Make sure you flush only the catheter and not the transducer. Be careful not to introduce any air.

The catheter is more likely to block whilst the balloon is inflated. For this reason flush the catheter after each reading. If the trace does become damped it is important to try to clear it as soon as possible otherwise the catheter will become blocked.

(4) Positive End Expiratory Pressure (PEEP). Remember PEEP will add to the intra thoracic pressure and that PA and wedge recordings will be accordingly higher.

SECTION XI REFERENCES

Central venous pressure and Swan-Ganz catheter

1   Latimer RD. Central venous catheterisation. *Br J Hosp Med* 1971; **5**: 309.

2   Leader. Jugular venous pressure. *Br Med J* 1974; **4**: 367.

3   Leader. Swan-Ganz catheter. *Lancet* 1978; **2**: 357.

4   Maki DG, Goldman DA. Rhame FS. Infection control in intravenous therapy. *Ann Intern Med* 1973; **79**: 867.

5   Riordan JF, Walters G, McLay WD. The significance of central venous pressure and cardiac output measurements in shock. *Postgrad Med J* 1969; **45**: 506.

Index

Numbers in heavy type indicate main reference page.

287